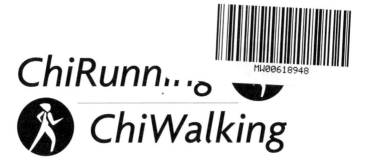

ChiRunning

ChiWalking

Daily Fitness Journal

From the bestselling authors of:

ChiRunning: A Revolutionary Approach to Effortless, Injury-Free Running

ChiWalking: Fitness Walking for Lifelong Health and Energy

Katherine and Danny Dreyer

ChiLiving, Inc.®
30 Orchard St.
Asheville, North Carolina 28801

Medical Disclaimer

This publication contains the opinions and ideas of its authors. It is sold with
the understanding that the authors and publisher are not engaged in rendering
exercise or health services in this book. The reader should consult his or her own
medical and health providers as appropriate before adopting any of the exercise
programs and suggestions in this book or drawing inferences from them.

The authors and publisher specifically disclaim all responsibility for any liability,
loss or risk, personal or otherwise, which is incurred as a consequence, directly
or indirectly, of the use and application of any of the contents of this book.

Please use caution and be sure to consult with a health care practitioner before
starting any physical fitness program. If you have any current mitigating heath-
related factors that you should consider as you begin a regular exercise program,
make an appointment to see your health care practitioner to get a thorough
physical exam and address any health concerns you may have.

Designed by Sean David Robinson
Edited by Elizabeth Frost and Shelly Schmidt
www.ChiRunning.com
www.ChiWalking.com
www.ChiLiving.com

DAILY FITNESS JOURNAL

Make a Choice:
Keep a Log, Achieve Your Goals

Making positive choices is key to maintaining a fitness program that works for you. Whether you're exercising for overall good health or preparing for a competitive event, keeping a log of your daily activity is the best way to establish and meet goals, track your progress and remember important information. The act of writing will help you clarify and solve problems so that you can make wise, informed decisions about your fitness program.

Inside, you'll find ample space to keep track of your thoughts and stats. There are also inspiring quotes, tips and pictures to keep you motivated.

ChiRunning and ChiWalking

Chi Running and Chi Walking tap into the powerful principles of T'ai Chi to create highly efficient, injury-free movement. This log can be used by anyone, at any time of year, and is particularly designed to support your Chi Running or Chi Walking practice. To learn more about these techniques, we suggest you read the books, watch the DVDs or find out more at ChiRunning.com.

Using this Log
This log provides space for you to:
- **Write** your Vision, Goals and Personal Assessments (Appendix A)
- **Plan** your month or your training program in weekly increments
- **Record** daily workout details
- **Review** your week and make positive choices for the next week
- **Graph** your progress of mileage, weight and Time Trial (Appendix B)
- **Keep** records of your races and events (Appendix E)

Know Yourself: Vision, Goals & Assessments

Appendix A is a place for you to write a vision for your personal success and specific goals you would like to accomplish. Your vision and goals create a powerful magnet that pull you toward your desired outcomes and can keep you motivated when challenges arise. Take the time to fill out the personal assessments as well. When you know your strengths and your vulnerabilities you will move forward with greater wisdom.

Monthly Overview & Weekly Planning

This log is organized by month, with a blank calendar at the beginning of each month, and on the opposing page there is space to write down your weekly goals.

SUN	MON	TUE	WED	THU	FRI	SAT
			(A)			

Dates: _____ (B)
Training Week #:
Weekly Goal:

Focus/Lesson:

Dates: _____ (C)
Training Week #:
Weekly Goal:

Focus/Lesson:

Dates:
Training Week #:
Weekly Goal: _____ (D)

Focus/Lesson:

Dates:
Training Week #:
Weekly Goal:

Focus/Lesson:

"Let him who would move the world first move himself."

– Socrates

© ChiLiving, Inc.

(A) **Monthly Calendar:** Feel free to write in important dates, training runs or events.

(B) **Training Week #:** Training for an event? Write down which training week you're in.

Ⓒ **Weekly Goal**: Set your goal for the week. Some suggestions:
- complete all workouts
- walk with a friend
- lower my PRE while running the same pace
- feel pelvic rotation at slower speeds

Ⓓ **Focus/Lesson**: Choose a focus or a lesson that needs your attention and concentrate on that for the week.

Weekly and Daily Workout Details

Each week begins on Monday and ends Sunday. In addition to daily logging fields, we incorporated space to include your current training phase, and if applicable, training week number, as well as an End-of-Week Review to help you assess your weekly progress.

What "Training Phase" are you in?

To maximize your workouts, it is always good to know what phase of training you're in. For example, if you are a beginner working on technique, you'd be in a Technique Phase. In the Chi Running & Chi Walking Training Programs, there are several phases of training: Vision & Planning, Technique, Conditioning, Event Mastery, Taper Time, The Event, and Rest & Renewal.

You may want to create your own inspirational terms for such phases as "Summer Fun," "Winter Maintenance" or any terms that inspire and motivate you.

Note your current training phase on the left-hand page of each week.

Training Week #: Do you have an event planned?

If you are training for a specific event, note the training week number in the top left-hand page of each week.

Daily Workout Details

Each daily logging area includes five fields for recording: four areas for stats and data from your workout, and an extra field with ample space for you to include other thoughts, feelings and impressions.

Workout/Route: Keep notes of specific workout details (speed intervals, fun run/walk, etc.). You might also have a favorite route that you can include here.

Time/Mileage/Pace: This field is reserved for tracking how long, how far or how fast you walk or run.

Focuses: We highly encourage you to include all focuses you practice during your workouts in this field. Keeping track of your Chi Running and Chi Walking focuses develops your skill in overcoming any obstacles while you're exercising. In Appendix D, you'll find a comprehensive list of focuses.

PRE/Body Sense: Body Sensing is the communication path between your mind and your body. Your PRE (Perceived Rate of Exertion) is your Body Sense of how much of an effort you are making in any given moment. For each workout, write down a Body Sense of your workout and/or keep track of a specific PRE. The PRE scale is from 1-10, 1 being no effort at all, 10 being the most effort possible.

Notes: The place for you to write down anything you encountered during your workout: weather, physical limitations, workout buddies, and challenges or breakthroughs with your form. Use this space for insights or thoughts that arise during your workout.

End-of-Week Review

Total Mileage/Time: Add up your weekly totals, whether miles or minutes, and include them here.

Year-to-Date: Whether you're keeping track of miles or minutes, you can keep a cumulative total.

Weight/BMI: We recommend weighing yourself on a weekly basis, first thing in the morning. Body Mass Index (BMI), may be an important component of your health, and we have provided space to record it. To determine your BMI, use our BMI tool at ChiRunning.com.

Shoe A/Shoe B: It's a good idea to have two pairs of shoes you alternate, especially if you're logging a lot of miles. Keep track of the mileage of your shoes.

Make a Choice and Move Forward: Assess your workouts from the current week, choose focuses or goals for the upcoming week, and create your approach for the future. This is a chance to be mindful about your progress and create the conditions for your success. Some of the notes you keep here can be used in the Weekly Goal section of the monthly view.

Chart Your Progress

Appendix B is the place to graph essential exercise components: distance, weight and Time Trial (time or average pace per mile). At the end of each week, you can enter the specific numbers from your weekly data into the chart and graph your progress.

This chart will provide an excellent visual tool for you as you review your health, habits and progress.

Race and Event Records

Whether you compete in 5ks every weekend or race only occasionally, Appendix E is the perfect place to keep track of races and events and record essential data.

Sustainable Exercise:
Themes to remember

A sustainable exercise program, combined with proper nutrition, is the key to good health and vitality. Two principles used in Chi Running and Chi Walking that contribute to a lifelong practice of healthy movement are Gradual Progress, and Form/Distance/Speed.

Read more about these and other key principles of intelligent movement in the Chi Running and Chi Walking books.

Gradual Progress – This is the principle underlying any natural and healthy growth process. Gradual Progress asks you to be gentle with yourself, and allow yourself to always be a "beginner" and discover the fun of learning something new. Every workout is an opportunity to learn something new about your technique and about yourself.

Form/Distance/Speed – A healthy fitness program built on good biomechanics and technique will prevent injury and allow you to be active for the rest of your life. With good form, distance is the means by which you build your aerobic and cardio conditioning. Speed is the natural outcome of good form and a solid conditioning base and can add challenge and fun to your workouts and goals.

Items to Support Your Fitness Program

- Chi Running & Chi Walking books, DVDs & audio programs
- Various training programs to help you meet your fitness goals, from a 5k to a marathon
- Sports Watch and Metronome – Important training tools for our programs

These and other training and fitness accessories may be found online at ChiRunning.com or ChiWalking.com.

Move Forward with Confidence

We hope this log inspires you, whether you walk or run, are beginning a weight-release program, or are training for your 10th marathon. Writing down your progress, challenges and breakthroughs will help you create the conditions for your own personal success.

Best wishes,
Katherine and Danny Dreyer and the ChiLiving Team

SUN	MON	TUE	WED	THU	FRI	SAT

"The secret of getting ahead is getting started."

– Sally Berger

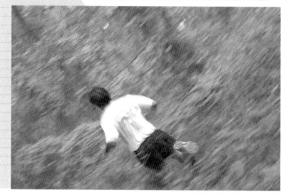

Dates:

Training Week #:

Weekly Goal:

Focus/Lesson:

Dates:

Training Week #:

Weekly Goal:

Focus/Lesson:

Dates:

Training Week #:

Weekly Goal:

Focus/Lesson:

Dates:

Training Week #:

Weekly Goal:

Focus/Lesson:

Dates:

Training Week #:

Weekly Goal:

Focus/Lesson:

Current Phase _____ Training Week # _____

Monday
Workout/Route _____

Mileage/Time/Pace _____

Focuses _____

PRE/Body Sense _____

Notes _____

_____

Tuesday
Workout/Route _____

Mileage/Time/Pace _____

Focuses _____

PRE/Body Sense _____

Notes _____

_____

Wednesday
Workout/Route _____

Mileage/Time/Pace _____

Focuses _____

PRE/Body Sense _____

Notes _____

_____

Thursday
Workout/Route _____

Mileage/Time/Pace _____

Focuses _____

PRE/Body Sense _____

Notes _____

_____

Friday
Workout/Route _____

Mileage/Time/Pace _____

Focuses _____

PRE/Body Sense _____

Notes _____

_____

Tip:
Do a slow jog before any race for
at least 15 minutes and then stretch,
followed by three or four 5-second
accelerations to really loosen
up your legs.

Saturday
Workout/Route _____
Mileage/Time/Pace _____
Focuses _____
PRE/Body Sense _____
Notes _____
_____

Sunday
Workout/Route _____
Mileage/Time/Pace _____
Focuses _____
PRE/Body Sense _____
Notes _____
_____

End-of-Week Review
Total Mileage/Time _____ Year-to-Date _____
Weight/BMI _____ Shoe A _____ Shoe B _____
Make a Choice and Move Forward _____
_____
_____
_____

Current Phase_____Training Week #_____

Monday
Workout/Route_____

Mileage/Time/Pace_____

Focuses_____

PRE/Body Sense_____

Notes_____

_____

Tuesday
Workout/Route_____

Mileage/Time/Pace_____

Focuses_____

PRE/Body Sense_____

Notes_____

_____

Wednesday
Workout/Route_____

Mileage/Time/Pace_____

Focuses_____

PRE/Body Sense___   _____

Notes_____

_____

Thursday
Workout/Route_____

Mileage/Time/Pace_____

Focuses_____

PRE/Body Sense_____

Notes_____

_____

Friday
Workout/Route_____

Mileage/Time/Pace_____

Focuses_____

PRE/Body Sense_____

Notes_____

_____

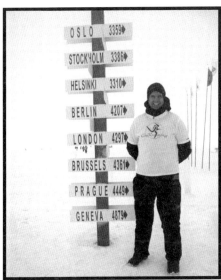

© ChiLiving, Inc.

Saturday
Workout/Route _____
Mileage/Time/Pace _____
Focuses _____
PRE/Body Sense _____
Notes _____
_____

Sunday
Workout/Route _____
Mileage/Time/Pace _____
Focuses _____
PRE/Body Sense _____
Notes _____
_____

End-of-Week Review
Total Mileage/Time _____ Year-to-Date _____
Weight/BMI _____ Shoe A _____ Shoe B _____
Make a Choice and Move Forward _____
_____
_____
_____

Current Phase _____ Training Week # _____

Monday
Workout/Route _____
Mileage/Time/Pace _____
Focuses _____
PRE/Body Sense _____
Notes _____
_____

Tuesday
Workout/Route _____
Mileage/Time/Pace _____
Focuses _____
PRE/Body Sense _____
Notes _____
_____

Wednesday
Workout/Route _____
Mileage/Time/Pace _____
Focuses _____
PRE/Body Sense _____
Notes _____
_____

Thursday
Workout/Route _____
Mileage/Time/Pace _____
Focuses _____
PRE/Body Sense _____
Notes _____
_____

Friday
Workout/Route _____
Mileage/Time/Pace _____
Focuses _____
PRE/Body Sense _____
Notes _____
_____

Tip:
If you feel tired when running or walking longer distances, shorten your stride length and engage your y'chi.

Saturday
Workout/Route _____
Mileage/Time/Pace _____
Focuses _____
PRE/Body Sense _____
Notes _____
_____

Sunday
Workout/Route _____
Mileage/Time/Pace _____
Focuses _____
PRE/Body Sense _____
Notes _____
_____

End-of-Week Review
Total Mileage/Time _____ Year-to-Date _____
Weight/BMI _____ Shoe A _____ Shoe B _____
Make a Choice and Move Forward _____
_____
_____

Current Phase_____Training Week #_____

Monday
Workout/Route_____
Mileage/Time/Pace_____
Focuses_____
PRE/Body Sense_____
Notes_____
_____

Tuesday
Workout/Route_____
Mileage/Time/Pace_____
Focuses_____
PRE/Body Sense_____
Notes_____
_____

Wednesday
Workout/Route_____
Mileage/Time/Pace_____
Focuses_____
PRE/Body Sense_____
Notes_____
_____

Thursday
Workout/Route_____
Mileage/Time/Pace_____
Focuses_____
PRE/Body Sense_____
Notes_____
_____

Friday
Workout/Route_____
Mileage/Time/Pace_____
Focuses_____
PRE/Body Sense_____
Notes_____
_____

> "Happiness is not a matter of intensity but of balance, order, rhythm and harmony."
>
> – *Thomas Morton*

Saturday

Workout/Route _____

Mileage/Time/Pace _____

Focuses _____

PRE/Body Sense _____

Notes _____

_____

Sunday

Workout/Route _____

Mileage/Time/Pace _____

Focuses _____

PRE/Body Sense _____

Notes _____

_____

End-of-Week Review

Total Mileage/Time _____ Year-to-Date _____

Weight/BMI _____ Shoe A _____ Shoe B _____

Make a Choice and Move Forward _____

_____

_____

_____

Current Phase _____ Training Week # _____

Monday
Workout/Route _____
Mileage/Time/Pace _____
Focuses _____
PRE/Body Sense _____
Notes _____

_____

Tuesday
Workout/Route _____
Mileage/Time/Pace _____
Focuses _____
PRE/Body Sense _____
Notes _____

_____

Wednesday
Workout/Route _____
Mileage/Time/Pace _____
Focuses _____
PRE/Body Sense _____
Notes _____

_____

Thursday
Workout/Route _____
Mileage/Time/Pace _____
Focuses _____
PRE/Body Sense _____
Notes _____

_____

Friday
Workout/Route _____
Mileage/Time/Pace _____
Focuses _____
PRE/Body Sense _____
Notes _____

_____

Month _____ **Week** _____

> "Impossibilities are merely things
> which we have not yet learned."
> – *Charles W. Chestnut*

Saturday
Workout/Route _____

Mileage/Time/Pace _____

Focuses _____

PRE/Body Sense _____

Notes _____

_____

Sunday
Workout/Route _____

Mileage/Time/Pace _____

Focuses _____

PRE/Body Sense _____

Notes _____

_____

End-of-Week Review
Total Mileage/Time _____ Year-to-Date _____

Weight/BMI _____ Shoe A _____ Shoe B _____

Make a Choice and Move Forward _____

_____

_____

SUN	MON	TUE	WED	THU	FRI	SAT

"Let him who would move the world first move himself."

– Socrates

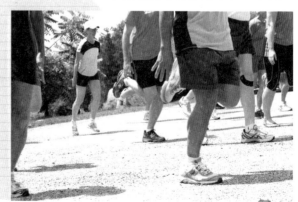

Dates:

Training Week #:

Weekly Goal:

Focus/Lesson:

Dates:

Training Week #:

Weekly Goal:

Focus/Lesson:

Dates:

Training Week #:

Weekly Goal:

Focus/Lesson:

Dates:

Training Week #:

Weekly Goal:

Focus/Lesson:

Dates:

Training Week #:

Weekly Goal:

Focus/Lesson:

Current Phase _____ Training Week # _____

Monday
Workout/Route _____
Mileage/Time/Pace _____
Focuses _____
PRE/Body Sense _____
Notes _____

_____

Tuesday
Workout/Route _____
Mileage/Time/Pace _____
Focuses _____
PRE/Body Sense _____
Notes _____

_____

Wednesday
Workout/Route _____
Mileage/Time/Pace _____
Focuses _____
PRE/Body Sense _____
Notes _____

_____

Thursday
Workout/Route _____
Mileage/Time/Pace _____
Focuses _____
PRE/Body Sense _____
Notes _____

_____

Friday
Workout/Route _____
Mileage/Time/Pace _____
Focuses _____
PRE/Body Sense _____
Notes _____

_____

Tip:

Make gravity do the work: Let your Column fall from your ankles and let gravity pull you forward, taking some of the work away from your tired legs. Remember not to bend at the waist!

Saturday

Workout/Route _____

Mileage/Time/Pace _____

Focuses _____

PRE/Body Sense _____

Notes _____

_____

Sunday

Workout/Route _____

Mileage/Time/Pace _____

Focuses _____

PRE/Body Sense _____

Notes _____

_____

End-of-Week Review

Total Mileage/Time _____ Year-to-Date _____

Weight/BMI _____ Shoe A _____ Shoe B _____

Make a Choice and Move Forward _____

_____

_____

_____

Current Phase_____Training Week #_____

Monday
Workout/Route_____
Mileage/Time/Pace_____
Focuses_____
PRE/Body Sense_____
Notes_____
_____

Tuesday
Workout/Route_____
Mileage/Time/Pace_____
Focuses_____
PRE/Body Sense_____
Notes_____
_____

Wednesday
Workout/Route_____
Mileage/Time/Pace_____
Focuses_____
PRE/Body Sense_____
Notes_____
_____

Thursday
Workout/Route_____
Mileage/Time/Pace_____
Focuses_____
PRE/Body Sense_____
Notes_____
_____

Friday
Workout/Route_____
Mileage/Time/Pace_____
Focuses_____
PRE/Body Sense_____
Notes_____
_____

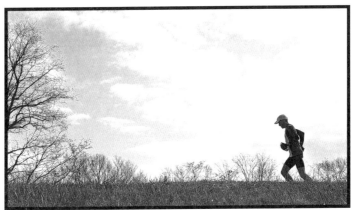

© Mark C.

Saturday
Workout/Route _____
Mileage/Time/Pace _____
Focuses _____
PRE/Body Sense _____
Notes _____
_____

Sunday
Workout/Route _____
Mileage/Time/Pace _____
Focuses _____
PRE/Body Sense _____
Notes _____
_____

End-of-Week Review
Total Mileage/Time _____ Year-to-Date _____
Weight/BMI _____ Shoe A _____ Shoe B _____
Make a Choice and Move Forward _____
_____
_____
_____

Current Phase _____ Training Week # _____

Monday
Workout/Route _____
Mileage/Time/Pace _____
Focuses _____
PRE/Body Sense _____
Notes _____

_____
_____

Tuesday
Workout/Route _____
Mileage/Time/Pace _____
Focuses _____
PRE/Body Sense _____
Notes _____

_____
_____

Wednesday
Workout/Route _____
Mileage/Time/Pace _____
Focuses _____
PRE/Body Sense _____
Notes _____

_____
_____

Thursday
Workout/Route _____
Mileage/Time/Pace _____
Focuses _____
PRE/Body Sense _____
Notes _____

_____
_____

Friday
Workout/Route _____
Mileage/Time/Pace _____
Focuses _____
PRE/Body Sense _____
Notes _____

_____
_____

> "You can only grow if you're willing to feel awkward and uncomfortable when you try something new."
> – *Brian Tracy*

Saturday
Workout/Route _____
Mileage/Time/Pace _____
Focuses _____
PRE/Body Sense _____
Notes _____
_____

Sunday
Workout/Route _____
Mileage/Time/Pace _____
Focuses _____
PRE/Body Sense _____
Notes _____
_____

End-of-Week Review
Total Mileage/Time _____ Year-to-Date _____
Weight/BMI _____ Shoe A _____ Shoe B _____
Make a Choice and Move Forward _____
_____
_____

Current Phase_____Training Week #_____

Monday
Workout/Route_____
Mileage/Time/Pace_____
Focuses_____
PRE/Body Sense_____
Notes_____
_____

Tuesday
Workout/Route_____
Mileage/Time/Pace_____
Focuses_____
PRE/Body Sense_____
Notes_____
_____

Wednesday
Workout/Route_____
Mileage/Time/Pace_____
Focuses_____
PRE/Body Sense_____
Notes_____
_____

Thursday
Workout/Route_____
Mileage/Time/Pace_____
Focuses_____
PRE/Body Sense_____
Notes_____
_____

Friday
Workout/Route_____
Mileage/Time/Pace_____
Focuses_____
PRE/Body Sense_____
Notes_____
_____

Tip:
Never step past your knee!

Saturday
Workout/Route _____
Mileage/Time/Pace _____
Focuses _____
PRE/Body Sense _____
Notes _____
_____

Sunday
Workout/Route _____
Mileage/Time/Pace _____
Focuses _____
PRE/Body Sense _____
Notes _____
_____

End-of-Week Review
Total Mileage/Time _____Year-to-Date _____
Weight/BMI _____ Shoe A _____ Shoe B _____
Make a Choice and Move Forward _____
_____
_____
_____

Current Phase _____ Training Week # _____

Monday
Workout/Route _____
Mileage/Time/Pace _____
Focuses _____
PRE/Body Sense _____
Notes _____

_____

Tuesday
Workout/Route _____
Mileage/Time/Pace _____
Focuses _____
PRE/Body Sense _____
Notes _____

_____

Wednesday
Workout/Route _____
Mileage/Time/Pace _____
Focuses _____
PRE/Body Sense _____
Notes _____

_____

Thursday
Workout/Route _____
Mileage/Time/Pace _____
Focuses _____
PRE/Body Sense _____
Notes _____

_____

Friday
Workout/Route _____
Mileage/Time/Pace _____
Focuses _____
PRE/Body Sense _____
Notes _____

_____

Month _____ Week _____

Tip:
Vary your pace while training. Pick up your pace at regular intervals, like every 1/2 hour. This will help circulate the lactic acid out of your legs and keep them from cramping or getting stiff.

Saturday
Workout/Route _____
Mileage/Time/Pace _____
Focuses _____
PRE/Body Sense _____
Notes _____
_____

Sunday
Workout/Route _____
Mileage/Time/Pace _____
Focuses _____
PRE/Body Sense _____
Notes _____
_____

End-of-Week Review
Total Mileage/Time _____ Year-to-Date _____
Weight/BMI _____ Shoe A _____ Shoe B _____
Make a Choice and Move Forward _____
_____
_____
_____
_____

SUN	MON	TUE	WED	THU	FRI	SAT

"No valid plans can be made by those who have no capacity for living now."

– Alan Watts

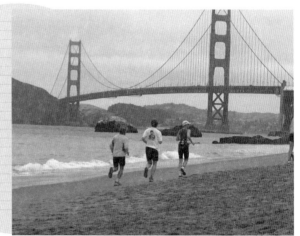

Dates:

Training Week #:

Weekly Goal:

Focus/Lesson:

Dates:

Training Week #:

Weekly Goal:

Focus/Lesson:

Dates:

Training Week #:

Weekly Goal:

Focus/Lesson:

Dates:

Training Week #:

Weekly Goal:

Focus/Lesson:

Dates:

Training Week #:

Weekly Goal:

Focus/Lesson:

Current Phase _____ Training Week # _____

Monday
Workout/Route _____
Mileage/Time/Pace _____
Focuses _____
PRE/Body Sense _____
Notes _____
_____

Tuesday
Workout/Route _____
Mileage/Time/Pace _____
Focuses _____
PRE/Body Sense _____
Notes _____
_____

Wednesday
Workout/Route _____
Mileage/Time/Pace _____
Focuses _____
PRE/Body Sense _____
Notes _____
_____

Thursday
Workout/Route _____
Mileage/Time/Pace _____
Focuses _____
PRE/Body Sense _____
Notes _____
_____

Friday
Workout/Route _____
Mileage/Time/Pace _____
Focuses _____
PRE/Body Sense _____
Notes _____
_____

Month ____ Week ____

Tip:
It takes about 25-30 miles to "break in" most running shoes. If you need new shoes for a race, give yourself at least 3 weeks to break them in.

Saturday
Workout/Route _____
Mileage/Time/Pace _____
Focuses _____
PRE/Body Sense _____
Notes _____

Sunday
Workout/Route _____
Mileage/Time/Pace _____
Focuses _____
PRE/Body Sense _____
Notes _____

End-of-Week Review
Total Mileage/Time _____ Year-to-Date _____
Weight/BMI _____ Shoe A _____ Shoe B _____
Make a Choice and Move Forward _____

Current Phase_____Training Week #_____

Monday
Workout/Route_____
Mileage/Time/Pace_____
Focuses_____
PRE/Body Sense_____
Notes_____

_____

Tuesday
Workout/Route_____
Mileage/Time/Pace_____
Focuses_____
PRE/Body Sense_____
Notes_____

_____

Wednesday
Workout/Route_____
Mileage/Time/Pace_____
Focuses_____
PRE/Body Sense_____
Notes_____

_____

Thursday
Workout/Route_____
Mileage/Time/Pace_____
Focuses_____
PRE/Body Sense_____
Notes_____

_____

Friday
Workout/Route_____
Mileage/Time/Pace_____
Focuses_____
PRE/Body Sense_____
Notes_____

_____

Month _____ Week _____

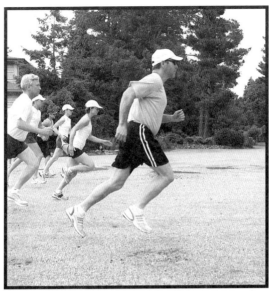

© ChiLiving, Inc.

Saturday

Workout/Route——————————————————————————————
Mileage/Time/Pace—————————————————————————————
Focuses——————————————————————————————————
PRE/Body Sense————————————————————————————————
Notes——————————————————————————————————————

Sunday

Workout/Route——————————————————————————————
Mileage/Time/Pace—————————————————————————————
Focuses——————————————————————————————————
PRE/Body Sense————————————————————————————————
Notes——————————————————————————————————————

End-of-Week Review

Total Mileage/Time——————————————Year-to-Date—————————
Weight/BMI————————————————— Shoe A——————— Shoe B———————
Make a Choice and Move Forward————————————————————————

Current Phase_____Training Week #_____

Monday
Workout/Route_____
Mileage/Time/Pace_____
Focuses_____
PRE/Body Sense_____
Notes_____
_____
_____

Tuesday
Workout/Route_____
Mileage/Time/Pace_____
Focuses_____
PRE/Body Sense_____
Notes_____
_____
_____

Wednesday
Workout/Route_____
Mileage/Time/Pace_____
Focuses_____
PRE/Body Sense_____
Notes_____
_____
_____

Thursday
Workout/Route_____
Mileage/Time/Pace_____
Focuses_____
PRE/Body Sense_____
Notes_____
_____
_____

Friday
Workout/Route_____
Mileage/Time/Pace_____
Focuses_____
PRE/Body Sense_____
Notes_____
_____
_____

Tip:
Imagine the earth is moving under you. You are moving along the world's largest treadmill.

Saturday
Workout/Route _____
Mileage/Time/Pace _____
Focuses _____
PRE/Body Sense _____
Notes _____
_____

Sunday
Workout/Route _____
Mileage/Time/Pace _____
Focuses _____
PRE/Body Sense _____
Notes _____
_____

End-of-Week Review
Total Mileage/Time _____ Year-to-Date _____
Weight/BMI _____ Shoe A _____ Shoe B _____
Make a Choice and Move Forward _____
_____
_____
_____

Current Phase _____ Training Week # _____

Monday
Workout/Route _____
Mileage/Time/Pace _____
Focuses _____
PRE/Body Sense _____
Notes _____
_____

Tuesday
Workout/Route _____
Mileage/Time/Pace _____
Focuses _____
PRE/Body Sense _____
Notes _____
_____

Wednesday
Workout/Route _____
Mileage/Time/Pace _____
Focuses _____
PRE/Body Sense _____
Notes _____
_____

Thursday
Workout/Route _____
Mileage/Time/Pace _____
Focuses _____
PRE/Body Sense _____
Notes _____
_____

Friday
Workout/Route _____
Mileage/Time/Pace _____
Focuses _____
PRE/Body Sense _____
Notes _____
_____

> "Obstacles are those frightful things you see when you take your eyes off your goal."
> – Henry Ford

Saturday
Workout/Route _____
Mileage/Time/Pace _____
Focuses _____
PRE/Body Sense _____
Notes _____

Sunday
Workout/Route _____
Mileage/Time/Pace _____
Focuses _____
PRE/Body Sense _____
Notes _____

End-of-Week Review
Total Mileage/Time _____ Year-to-Date _____
Weight/BMI _____ Shoe A _____ Shoe B _____
Make a Choice and Move Forward _____

Current Phase _____ Training Week # _____

Monday
Workout/Route _____
Mileage/Time/Pace _____
Focuses _____
PRE/Body Sense _____
Notes _____

_____

Tuesday
Workout/Route _____
Mileage/Time/Pace _____
Focuses _____
PRE/Body Sense _____
Notes _____

_____

Wednesday
Workout/Route _____
Mileage/Time/Pace _____
Focuses _____
PRE/Body Sense _____
Notes _____

_____

Thursday
Workout/Route _____
Mileage/Time/Pace _____
Focuses _____
PRE/Body Sense _____
Notes _____

_____

Friday
Workout/Route _____
Mileage/Time/Pace _____
Focuses _____
PRE/Body Sense _____
Notes _____

_____

Month _____ Week _____

> "Let us not look back in anger, nor forward in fear, but around in awareness."
> – James Thurber

Saturday
Workout/Route _____
Mileage/Time/Pace _____
Focuses _____
PRE/Body Sense _____
Notes _____
_____

Sunday
Workout/Route _____
Mileage/Time/Pace _____
Focuses _____
PRE/Body Sense _____
Notes _____
_____

End-of-Week Review
Total Mileage/Time _____ Year-to-Date _____
Weight/BMI _____ Shoe A _____ Shoe B _____
Make a Choice and Move Forward _____
_____
_____
_____

SUN	MON	TUE	WED	THU	FRI	SAT

"Man cannot discover new oceans unless he has the courage to lose sight of the shore."

– Andre Gide

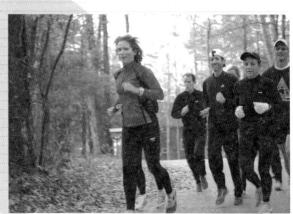

Dates:

Training Week #:

Weekly Goal:

Focus/Lesson:

Dates:

Training Week #:

Weekly Goal:

Focus/Lesson:

Dates:

Training Week #:

Weekly Goal:

Focus/Lesson:

Dates:

Training Week #:

Weekly Goal:

Focus/Lesson:

Dates:

Training Week #:

Weekly Goal:

Focus/Lesson:

Current Phase _____Training Week # _____

Monday

Workout/Route _____

Mileage/Time/Pace _____

Focuses _____

PRE/Body Sense _____

Notes _____

_____

Tuesday

Workout/Route _____

Mileage/Time/Pace _____

Focuses _____

PRE/Body Sense _____

Notes _____

_____

Wednesday

Workout/Route _____

Mileage/Time/Pace _____

Focuses _____

PRE/Body Sense _____

Notes _____

_____

Thursday

Workout/Route _____

Mileage/Time/Pace _____

Focuses _____

PRE/Body Sense _____

Notes _____

_____

Friday

Workout/Route _____

Mileage/Time/Pace _____

Focuses _____

PRE/Body Sense _____

Notes _____

_____

Saturday
Workout/Route _____
Mileage/Time/Pace _____
Focuses _____
PRE/Body Sense _____
Notes _____
_____

Sunday
Workout/Route _____
Mileage/Time/Pace _____
Focuses _____
PRE/Body Sense _____
Notes _____
_____

End-of-Week Review
Total Mileage/Time _____Year-to-Date _____
Weight/BMI _____ Shoe A _____ Shoe B _____
Make a Choice and Move Forward _____
_____
_____
_____

Current Phase _____ Training Week # _____

Monday
Workout/Route _____
Mileage/Time/Pace _____
Focuses _____
PRE/Body Sense _____
Notes _____

_____

Tuesday
Workout/Route _____
Mileage/Time/Pace _____
Focuses _____
PRE/Body Sense _____
Notes _____

_____

Wednesday
Workout/Route _____
Mileage/Time/Pace _____
Focuses _____
PRE/Body Sense _____
Notes _____

_____

Thursday
Workout/Route _____
Mileage/Time/Pace _____
Focuses _____
PRE/Body Sense _____
Notes _____

_____

Friday
Workout/Route _____
Mileage/Time/Pace _____
Focuses _____
PRE/Body Sense _____
Notes _____

_____

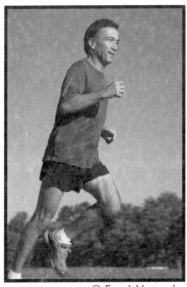

© Frank Veronsky

Saturday

Workout/Route
Mileage/Time/Pace
Focuses
PRE/Body Sense
Notes

Sunday

Workout/Route
Mileage/Time/Pace
Focuses
PRE/Body Sense
Notes

End-of-Week Review

Total Mileage/Time ————————————— Year-to-Date ————
Weight/BMI ——————————— Shoe A ———— Shoe B ————
Make a Choice and Move Forward

Current Phase _____ Training Week # _____

Monday
Workout/Route _____
Mileage/Time/Pace _____
Focuses _____
PRE/Body Sense _____
Notes _____
_____
_____

Tuesday
Workout/Route _____
Mileage/Time/Pace _____
Focuses _____
PRE/Body Sense _____
Notes _____
_____
_____

Wednesday
Workout/Route _____
Mileage/Time/Pace _____
Focuses _____
PRE/Body Sense _____
Notes _____
_____
_____

Thursday
Workout/Route _____
Mileage/Time/Pace _____
Focuses _____
PRE/Body Sense _____
Notes _____
_____
_____

Friday
Workout/Route _____
Mileage/Time/Pace _____
Focuses _____
PRE/Body Sense _____
Notes _____
_____
_____

Tip:
Non-identification is the practice of
putting your ego away,
and accepting things for what
they truly are.

Saturday
Workout/Route _____
Mileage/Time/Pace _____
Focuses _____
PRE/Body Sense _____
Notes _____
_____
_____

Sunday
Workout/Route _____
Mileage/Time/Pace _____
Focuses _____
PRE/Body Sense _____
Notes _____
_____
_____

End-of-Week Review
Total Mileage/Time _____ Year-to-Date _____
Weight/BMI _____ Shoe A _____ Shoe B _____
Make a Choice and Move Forward _____
_____
_____
_____
_____

Current Phase _____ Training Week # _____

Monday
Workout/Route _____

Mileage/Time/Pace _____

Focuses _____

PRE/Body Sense _____

Notes _____

_____

Tuesday
Workout/Route _____

Mileage/Time/Pace _____

Focuses _____

PRE/Body Sense _____

Notes _____

_____

Wednesday
Workout/Route _____

Mileage/Time/Pace _____

Focuses _____

PRE/Body Sense _____

Notes _____

_____

Thursday
Workout/Route _____

Mileage/Time/Pace _____

Focuses _____

PRE/Body Sense _____

Notes _____

_____

Friday
Workout/Route _____

Mileage/Time/Pace _____

Focuses _____

PRE/Body Sense _____

Notes _____

_____

> "The impossible is
> often the untried."
> – Jim Goodwin

Saturday
Workout/Route _____
Mileage/Time/Pace _____
Focuses _____
PRE/Body Sense _____
Notes _____
_____

Sunday
Workout/Route _____
Mileage/Time/Pace _____
Focuses _____
PRE/Body Sense _____
Notes _____
_____

End-of-Week Review
Total Mileage/Time _____ Year-to-Date _____
Weight/BMI _____ Shoe A _____ Shoe B _____
Make a Choice and Move Forward _____
_____
_____
_____

Current Phase _____ Training Week # _____

Monday
Workout/Route _____

Mileage/Time/Pace _____

Focuses _____

PRE/Body Sense _____

Notes _____

_____

_____

Tuesday
Workout/Route _____

Mileage/Time/Pace _____

Focuses _____

PRE/Body Sense _____

Notes _____

_____

_____

Wednesday
Workout/Route _____

Mileage/Time/Pace _____

Focuses _____

PRE/Body Sense _____

Notes _____

_____

_____

Thursday
Workout/Route _____

Mileage/Time/Pace _____

Focuses _____

PRE/Body Sense _____

Notes _____

_____

_____

Friday
Workout/Route _____

Mileage/Time/Pace _____

Focuses _____

PRE/Body Sense _____

Notes _____

_____

Month _____ Week _____

> "The greatest mistake you can make
> in life is to be continually fearing you
> will make one."
> – *Elbert Hubbard*

Saturday
Workout/Route _____
Mileage/Time/Pace _____
Focuses _____
PRE/Body Sense _____
Notes _____
_____

Sunday
Workout/Route _____
Mileage/Time/Pace _____
Focuses _____
PRE/Body Sense _____
Notes _____
_____

End-of-Week Review
Total Mileage/Time _____Year-to-Date _____
Weight/BMI _____ Shoe A _____ Shoe B _____
Make a Choice and Move Forward _____
_____
_____
_____

SUN	MON	TUE	WED	THU	FRI	SAT

"Don't be afraid to go out on a limb. That's where the fruit is."

– H. Jackson Browne

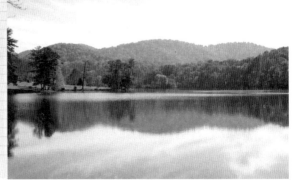

Dates:

Training Week #:

Weekly Goal:

Focus/Lesson:

Dates:

Training Week #:

Weekly Goal:

Focus/Lesson:

Dates:

Training Week #:

Weekly Goal:

Focus/Lesson:

Dates:

Training Week #:

Weekly Goal:

Focus/Lesson:

Dates:

Training Week #:

Weekly Goal:

Focus/Lesson:

Current Phase _____ Training Week # _____

Monday
Workout/Route _____
Mileage/Time/Pace _____
Focuses _____
PRE/Body Sense _____
Notes _____
_____

Tuesday
Workout/Route _____
Mileage/Time/Pace _____
Focuses _____
PRE/Body Sense _____
Notes _____
_____

Wednesday
Workout/Route _____
Mileage/Time/Pace _____
Focuses _____
PRE/Body Sense _____
Notes _____
_____

Thursday
Workout/Route _____
Mileage/Time/Pace _____
Focuses _____
PRE/Body Sense _____
Notes _____
_____

Friday
Workout/Route _____
Mileage/Time/Pace _____
Focuses _____
PRE/Body Sense _____
Notes _____
_____

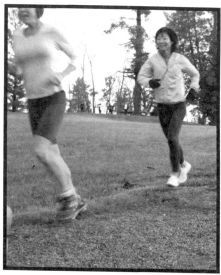

© ChiLiving, Inc.

Saturday

Workout/Route _____

Mileage/Time/Pace _____

Focuses _____

PRE/Body Sense _____

Notes _____

_____

Sunday

Workout/Route _____

Mileage/Time/Pace _____

Focuses _____

PRE/Body Sense _____

Notes _____

_____

End-of-Week Review

Total Mileage/Time _____ Year-to-Date _____

Weight/BMI _____ Shoe A _____ Shoe B _____

Make a Choice and Move Forward _____

_____

_____

_____

Current Phase _____ Training Week # _____

Monday

Workout/Route _____

Mileage/Time/Pace _____

Focuses _____

PRE/Body Sense _____

Notes _____

_____

Tuesday

Workout/Route _____

Mileage/Time/Pace _____

Focuses _____

PRE/Body Sense _____

Notes _____

_____

Wednesday

Workout/Route _____

Mileage/Time/Pace _____

Focuses _____

PRE/Body Sense _____

Notes _____

_____

Thursday

Workout/Route _____

Mileage/Time/Pace _____

Focuses _____

PRE/Body Sense _____

Notes _____

_____

Friday

Workout/Route _____

Mileage/Time/Pace _____

Focuses _____

PRE/Body Sense _____

Notes _____

_____

Tip:
Practice belly-breathing: It can energize, calm, cleanse and empower the body and the mind.

Saturday
Workout/Route _____
Mileage/Time/Pace _____
Focuses _____
PRE/Body Sense _____
Notes _____
_____

Sunday
Workout/Route _____
Mileage/Time/Pace _____
Focuses _____
PRE/Body Sense _____
Notes _____
_____

End-of-Week Review
Total Mileage/Time _____ Year-to-Date _____
Weight/BMI _____ Shoe A _____ Shoe B _____
Make a Choice and Move Forward _____
_____
_____
_____

Current Phase _____ Training Week # _____

Monday
Workout/Route _____
Mileage/Time/Pace _____
Focuses _____
PRE/Body Sense _____
Notes _____
_____

Tuesday
Workout/Route _____
Mileage/Time/Pace _____
Focuses _____
PRE/Body Sense _____
Notes _____
_____

Wednesday
Workout/Route _____
Mileage/Time/Pace _____
Focuses _____
PRE/Body Sense _____
Notes _____
_____

Thursday
Workout/Route _____
Mileage/Time/Pace _____
Focuses _____
PRE/Body Sense _____
Notes _____
_____

Friday
Workout/Route _____
Mileage/Time/Pace _____
Focuses _____
PRE/Body Sense _____
Notes _____
_____

> "The time to relax is when you don't have time for it."
> – *Sydney J. Harris*

Saturday
Workout/Route _____
Mileage/Time/Pace _____
Focuses _____
PRE/Body Sense _____
Notes _____
_____

Sunday
Workout/Route _____
Mileage/Time/Pace _____
Focuses _____
PRE/Body Sense _____
Notes _____
_____

End-of-Week Review
Total Mileage/Time _____ Year-to-Date _____
Weight/BMI _____ Shoe A _____ Shoe B _____
Make a Choice and Move Forward _____
_____
_____
_____

Current Phase_____Training Week #_____

Monday
Workout/Route_____
Mileage/Time/Pace_____
Focuses_____
PRE/Body Sense_____
Notes_____
_____

Tuesday
Workout/Route_____
Mileage/Time/Pace_____
Focuses_____
PRE/Body Sense_____
Notes_____
_____

Wednesday
Workout/Route_____
Mileage/Time/Pace_____
Focuses_____
PRE/Body Sense_____
Notes_____
_____

Thursday
Workout/Route_____
Mileage/Time/Pace_____
Focuses_____
PRE/Body Sense_____
Notes_____
_____

Friday
Workout/Route_____
Mileage/Time/Pace_____
Focuses_____
PRE/Body Sense_____
Notes_____
_____

Tip:
Engaging your core and finding
your inner balance go hand in hand.
One cannot happen without
the other.

Saturday
Workout/Route _____
Mileage/Time/Pace _____
Focuses _____
PRE/Body Sense _____
Notes _____

Sunday
Workout/Route _____
Mileage/Time/Pace _____
Focuses _____
PRE/Body Sense _____
Notes _____

End-of-Week Review
Total Mileage/Time _____Year-to-Date _____
Weight/BMI _____ Shoe A _____ Shoe B _____
Make a Choice and Move Forward _____
_____
_____
_____

Current Phase _____ Training Week # _____

Monday
Workout/Route _____
Mileage/Time/Pace _____
Focuses _____
PRE/Body Sense _____
Notes _____
_____

Tuesday
Workout/Route _____
Mileage/Time/Pace _____
Focuses _____
PRE/Body Sense _____
Notes _____
_____

Wednesday
Workout/Route _____
Mileage/Time/Pace _____
Focuses _____
PRE/Body Sense _____
Notes _____
_____

Thursday
Workout/Route _____
Mileage/Time/Pace _____
Focuses _____
PRE/Body Sense _____
Notes _____
_____

Friday
Workout/Route _____
Mileage/Time/Pace _____
Focuses _____
PRE/Body Sense _____
Notes _____
_____

Month _____ **Week** _____

Tip:

When running a 5K or a 10K, try to build up to running one 5K or 10K per week in training. Training your body for endurance is the best guarantee that you'll have a good run on race day.

Saturday

Workout/Route _____

Mileage/Time/Pace _____

Focuses _____

PRE/Body Sense _____

Notes _____

_____

Sunday

Workout/Route _____

Mileage/Time/Pace _____

Focuses _____

PRE/Body Sense _____

Notes _____

_____

End-of-Week Review

Total Mileage/Time _____ Year-to-Date _____

Weight/BMI _____ Shoe A _____ Shoe B _____

Make a Choice and Move Forward _____

_____

_____

_____

SUN	MON	TUE	WED	THU	FRI	SAT

"Our strength
grows out of our
weaknesses."

– Ralph Waldo
   Emerson

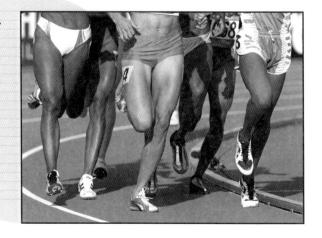

Dates:

Training Week #:

Weekly Goal:

Focus/Lesson:

Dates:

Training Week #:

Weekly Goal:

Focus/Lesson:

Dates:

Training Week #:

Weekly Goal:

Focus/Lesson:

Dates:

Training Week #:

Weekly Goal:

Focus/Lesson:

Dates:

Training Week #:

Weekly Goal:

Focus/Lesson:

Current Phase_____Training Week #_____

Monday
Workout/Route_____
Mileage/Time/Pace_____
Focuses_____
PRE/Body Sense_____
Notes_____
_____

Tuesday
Workout/Route_____
Mileage/Time/Pace_____
Focuses_____
PRE/Body Sense_____
Notes_____
_____

Wednesday
Workout/Route_____
Mileage/Time/Pace_____
Focuses_____
PRE/Body Sense_____
Notes_____
_____

Thursday
Workout/Route_____
Mileage/Time/Pace_____
Focuses_____
PRE/Body Sense_____
Notes_____
_____

Friday
Workout/Route_____
Mileage/Time/Pace_____
Focuses_____
PRE/Body Sense_____
Notes_____
_____

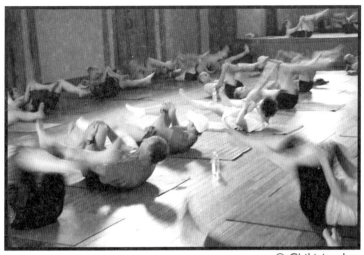

© ChiLiving, Inc.

Saturday

Workout/Route _____

Mileage/Time/Pace _____

Focuses _____

PRE/Body Sense _____

Notes _____

_____

Sunday

Workout/Route _____

Mileage/Time/Pace _____

Focuses _____

PRE/Body Sense _____

Notes _____

_____

End-of-Week Review

Total Mileage/Time _____ Year-to-Date _____

Weight/BMI _____ Shoe A _____ Shoe B _____

Make a Choice and Move Forward _____

_____

_____

_____

Current Phase_____Training Week #_____

Monday
Workout/Route_____
Mileage/Time/Pace_____
Focuses_____
PRE/Body Sense_____
Notes_____
_____

Tuesday
Workout/Route_____
Mileage/Time/Pace_____
Focuses_____
PRE/Body Sense_____
Notes_____
_____

Wednesday
Workout/Route_____
Mileage/Time/Pace_____
Focuses_____
PRE/Body Sense_____
Notes_____
_____

Thursday
Workout/Route_____
Mileage/Time/Pace_____
Focuses_____
PRE/Body Sense_____
Notes_____
_____

Friday
Workout/Route_____
Mileage/Time/Pace_____
Focuses_____
PRE/Body Sense_____
Notes_____
_____

Tip:
Splashy water at the aid stations?
When you grab a cup from a
volunteer, crimp the top so that only
a little water will come out through a
"spout" into your mouth!

Saturday
Workout/Route _____
Mileage/Time/Pace _____
Focuses _____
PRE/Body Sense _____
Notes _____
_____

Sunday
Workout/Route _____
Mileage/Time/Pace _____
Focuses _____
PRE/Body Sense _____
Notes _____
_____

End-of-Week Review
Total Mileage/Time _____ Year-to-Date _____
Weight/BMI _____ Shoe A _____ Shoe B _____
Make a Choice and Move Forward _____
_____
_____
_____

Current Phase _____Training Week # _____

Monday
Workout/Route _____
Mileage/Time/Pace _____
Focuses _____
PRE/Body Sense _____
Notes _____
_____

Tuesday
Workout/Route _____
Mileage/Time/Pace _____
Focuses _____
PRE/Body Sense _____
Notes _____
_____

Wednesday
Workout/Route _____
Mileage/Time/Pace _____
Focuses _____
PRE/Body Sense _____
Notes _____
_____

Thursday
Workout/Route _____
Mileage/Time/Pace _____
Focuses _____
PRE/Body Sense _____
Notes _____
_____

Friday
Workout/Route _____
Mileage/Time/Pace _____
Focuses _____
PRE/Body Sense _____
Notes _____
_____

Month _____ Week _____

> "It is easier to go down a hill
> than up, but the view
> is best from the top."
> – *Arnold Bennet*

Saturday
Workout/Route _____
Mileage/Time/Pace _____
Focuses _____
PRE/Body Sense _____
Notes _____
_____

Sunday
Workout/Route _____
Mileage/Time/Pace _____
Focuses _____
PRE/Body Sense _____
Notes _____
_____

End-of-Week Review
Total Mileage/Time _____Year-to-Date _____
Weight/BMI _____ Shoe A _____ Shoe B _____
Make a Choice and Move Forward _____
_____
_____
_____

Current Phase _____ Training Week # _____

Monday
Workout/Route _____
Mileage/Time/Pace _____
Focuses _____
PRE/Body Sense _____
Notes _____
_____

Tuesday
Workout/Route _____
Mileage/Time/Pace _____
Focuses _____
PRE/Body Sense _____
Notes _____
_____

Wednesday
Workout/Route _____
Mileage/Time/Pace _____
Focuses _____
PRE/Body Sense _____
Notes _____
_____

Thursday
Workout/Route _____
Mileage/Time/Pace _____
Focuses _____
PRE/Body Sense _____
Notes _____
_____

Friday
Workout/Route _____
Mileage/Time/Pace _____
Focuses _____
PRE/Body Sense _____
Notes _____
_____

> ## Tip:
> Remember to practice your y'chi:
> It is the ability to focus energy
> through your eyes.

Saturday

Workout/Route _____

Mileage/Time/Pace _____

Focuses _____

PRE/Body Sense _____

Notes _____

_____

Sunday

Workout/Route _____

Mileage/Time/Pace _____

Focuses _____

PRE/Body Sense _____

Notes _____

_____

End-of-Week Review

Total Mileage/Time _____ Year-to-Date _____

Weight/BMI _____ Shoe A _____ Shoe B _____

Make a Choice and Move Forward _____

_____

_____

_____

Current Phase_____Training Week #_____

Monday
Workout/Route_____
Mileage/Time/Pace_____
Focuses_____
PRE/Body Sense_____
Notes_____
_____

Tuesday
Workout/Route_____
Mileage/Time/Pace_____
Focuses_____
PRE/Body Sense_____
Notes_____
_____

Wednesday
Workout/Route_____
Mileage/Time/Pace_____
Focuses_____
PRE/Body Sense_____
Notes_____
_____

Thursday
Workout/Route_____
Mileage/Time/Pace_____
Focuses_____
PRE/Body Sense_____
Notes_____
_____

Friday
Workout/Route_____
Mileage/Time/Pace_____
Focuses_____
PRE/Body Sense_____
Notes_____
_____

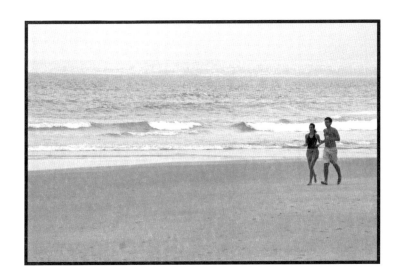

Saturday
Workout/Route _____

Mileage/Time/Pace _____

Focuses _____

PRE/Body Sense _____

Notes _____

_____

Sunday
Workout/Route _____

Mileage/Time/Pace _____

Focuses _____

PRE/Body Sense _____

Notes _____

_____

End-of-Week Review
Total Mileage/Time _____ Year-to-Date _____

Weight/BMI _____ Shoe A _____ Shoe B _____

Make a Choice and Move Forward _____

_____

_____

_____

SUN	MON	TUE	WED	THU	FRI	SAT

"Most people
run a race to see
who is fastest. I
run a race to see
who has the most
guts."

– Steve Prefontaine

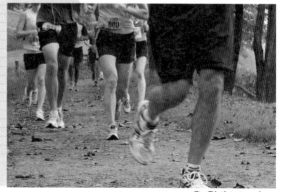

Dates:

Training Week #:

Weekly Goal:

Focus/Lesson:

Dates:

Training Week #:

Weekly Goal:

Focus/Lesson:

Dates:

Training Week #:

Weekly Goal:

Focus/Lesson:

Dates:

Training Week #:

Weekly Goal:

Focus/Lesson:

Dates:

Training Week #:

Weekly Goal:

Focus/Lesson:

Current Phase_____Training Week #_____

Monday
Workout/Route_____
Mileage/Time/Pace_____
Focuses_____
PRE/Body Sense_____
Notes_____

_____

Tuesday
Workout/Route_____
Mileage/Time/Pace_____
Focuses_____
PRE/Body Sense_____
Notes_____

_____

Wednesday
Workout/Route_____
Mileage/Time/Pace_____
Focuses_____
PRE/Body Sense_____
Notes_____

_____

Thursday
Workout/Route_____
Mileage/Time/Pace_____
Focuses_____
PRE/Body Sense_____
Notes_____

_____

Friday
Workout/Route_____
Mileage/Time/Pace_____
Focuses_____
PRE/Body Sense_____
Notes_____

_____

Tip:
Tired legs? Pretend you're shifting from 4th gear to 3rd gear, and increase your cadence while shortening your stride length.

Saturday
Workout/Route _____
Mileage/Time/Pace _____
Focuses _____
PRE/Body Sense _____
Notes _____
_____

Sunday
Workout/Route _____
Mileage/Time/Pace _____
Focuses _____
PRE/Body Sense _____
Notes _____
_____

End-of-Week Review
Total Mileage/Time _____ Year-to-Date _____
Weight/BMI _____ Shoe A _____ Shoe B _____
Make a Choice and Move Forward _____
_____
_____
_____

Current Phase_____Training Week #_____

Monday
Workout/Route_____
Mileage/Time/Pace_____
Focuses_____
PRE/Body Sense_____
Notes_____
_____

Tuesday
Workout/Route_____
Mileage/Time/Pace_____
Focuses_____
PRE/Body Sense_____
Notes_____
_____

Wednesday
Workout/Route_____
Mileage/Time/Pace_____
Focuses_____
PRE/Body Sense_____
Notes_____
_____

Thursday
Workout/Route_____
Mileage/Time/Pace_____
Focuses_____
PRE/Body Sense_____
Notes_____
_____

Friday
Workout/Route_____
Mileage/Time/Pace_____
Focuses_____
PRE/Body Sense_____
Notes_____
_____

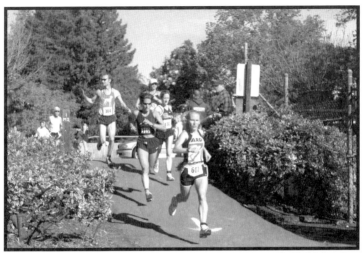

© ChiLiving, Inc.

Saturday

Workout/Route _____

Mileage/Time/Pace _____

Focuses _____

PRE/Body Sense _____

Notes _____

_____

Sunday

Workout/Route _____

Mileage/Time/Pace _____

Focuses _____

PRE/Body Sense _____

Notes _____

_____

End-of-Week Review

Total Mileage/Time _____ Year-to-Date _____

Weight/BMI _____ Shoe A _____ Shoe B _____

Make a Choice and Move Forward _____

_____

_____

Current Phase_____Training Week #_____

Monday
Workout/Route_____
Mileage/Time/Pace_____
Focuses_____
PRE/Body Sense_____
Notes_____
_____

Tuesday
Workout/Route_____
Mileage/Time/Pace_____
Focuses_____
PRE/Body Sense_____
Notes_____
_____

Wednesday
Workout/Route_____
Mileage/Time/Pace_____
Focuses_____
PRE/Body Sense_____
Notes_____
_____

Thursday
Workout/Route_____
Mileage/Time/Pace_____
Focuses_____
PRE/Body Sense_____
Notes_____
_____

Friday
Workout/Route_____
Mileage/Time/Pace_____
Focuses_____
PRE/Body Sense_____
Notes_____
_____

Tip:
On race day, eat lightly; bananas, toast and honey, fruits, dates or raisins and don't eat any new foods that you're not accustomed to.

Saturday
Workout/Route _____
Mileage/Time/Pace _____
Focuses _____
PRE/Body Sense _____
Notes _____

Sunday
Workout/Route _____
Mileage/Time/Pace _____
Focuses _____
PRE/Body Sense _____
Notes _____

End-of-Week Review
Total Mileage/Time _____ Year-to-Date _____
Weight/BMI _____ Shoe A _____ Shoe B _____
Make a Choice and Move Forward _____

Current Phase _____ Training Week # _____

Monday
Workout/Route _____
Mileage/Time/Pace _____
Focuses _____
PRE/Body Sense _____
Notes _____

_____

Tuesday
Workout/Route _____
Mileage/Time/Pace _____
Focuses _____
PRE/Body Sense _____
Notes _____

_____

Wednesday
Workout/Route _____
Mileage/Time/Pace _____
Focuses _____
PRE/Body Sense _____
Notes _____

_____

Thursday
Workout/Route _____
Mileage/Time/Pace _____
Focuses _____
PRE/Body Sense _____
Notes _____

_____

Friday
Workout/Route _____
Mileage/Time/Pace _____
Focuses _____
PRE/Body Sense _____
Notes _____

_____

> "Aerodynamically, the bumblebee shouldn't be able to fly, but the bumblebee doesn't know that, so it goes on flying anyway"
> – *Mary Kay Ash*

Saturday
Workout/Route _____
Mileage/Time/Pace _____
Focuses _____
PRE/Body Sense _____
Notes _____
_____

Sunday
Workout/Route _____
Mileage/Time/Pace _____
Focuses _____
PRE/Body Sense _____
Notes _____
_____

End-of-Week Review
Total Mileage/Time _____ Year-to-Date _____
Weight/BMI _____ Shoe A _____ Shoe B _____
Make a Choice and Move Forward _____
_____
_____
_____

Current Phase _____ Training Week # _____

Monday
Workout/Route _____
Mileage/Time/Pace _____
Focuses _____
PRE/Body Sense _____
Notes _____
_____

Tuesday
Workout/Route _____
Mileage/Time/Pace _____
Focuses _____
PRE/Body Sense _____
Notes _____
_____

Wednesday
Workout/Route _____
Mileage/Time/Pace _____
Focuses _____
PRE/Body Sense _____
Notes _____
_____

Thursday
Workout/Route _____
Mileage/Time/Pace _____
Focuses _____
PRE/Body Sense _____
Notes _____
_____

Friday
Workout/Route _____
Mileage/Time/Pace _____
Focuses _____
PRE/Body Sense _____
Notes _____
_____

Tip:
When racing, stay relaxed at the start and you'll do much better at the finish.

Saturday
Workout/Route _____
Mileage/Time/Pace _____
Focuses _____
PRE/Body Sense _____
Notes _____
_____

Sunday
Workout/Route _____
Mileage/Time/Pace _____
Focuses _____
PRE/Body Sense _____
Notes _____
_____

End-of-Week Review
Total Mileage/Time _____ Year-to-Date _____
Weight/BMI _____ Shoe A _____ Shoe B _____
Make a Choice and Move Forward _____
_____
_____
_____

SUN	MON	TUE	WED	THU	FRI	SAT

"Commitment
leads to action.
Action brings
your dream
closer."

– Marcia Wieder

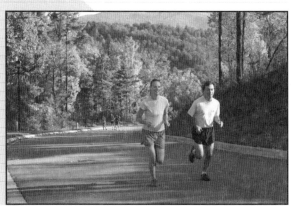

Dates:

Training Week #:

Weekly Goal:

Focus/Lesson:

Dates:

Training Week #:

Weekly Goal:

Focus/Lesson:

Dates:

Training Week #:

Weekly Goal:

Focus/Lesson:

Dates:

Training Week #:

Weekly Goal:

Focus/Lesson:

Dates:

Training Week #:

Weekly Goal:

Focus/Lesson:

Current Phase _____ Training Week # _____

Monday
Workout/Route _____
Mileage/Time/Pace _____
Focuses _____
PRE/Body Sense _____
Notes _____

_____
_____

Tuesday
Workout/Route _____
Mileage/Time/Pace _____
Focuses _____
PRE/Body Sense _____
Notes _____

_____
_____

Wednesday
Workout/Route _____
Mileage/Time/Pace _____
Focuses _____
PRE/Body Sense _____
Notes _____

_____
_____

Thursday
Workout/Route _____
Mileage/Time/Pace _____
Focuses _____
PRE/Body Sense _____
Notes _____

_____
_____

Friday
Workout/Route _____
Mileage/Time/Pace _____
Focuses _____
PRE/Body Sense _____
Notes _____

_____
_____

Tip:
Race day? Drink 18-24 oz. of water at least 2 hours before the race. During the race you should take a sip of water every 10 minutes.

Saturday
Workout/Route _____

Mileage/Time/Pace _____

Focuses _____

PRE/Body Sense _____

Notes _____

_____

Sunday
Workout/Route _____

Mileage/Time/Pace _____

Focuses _____

PRE/Body Sense _____

Notes _____

_____

End-of-Week Review
Total Mileage/Time _____ Year-to-Date _____

Weight/BMI _____ Shoe A _____ Shoe B _____

Make a Choice and Move Forward _____

_____

_____

_____

Current Phase_____Training Week #_____

Monday
Workout/Route_____
Mileage/Time/Pace_____
Focuses_____
PRE/Body Sense_____
Notes_____

_____

Tuesday
Workout/Route_____
Mileage/Time/Pace_____
Focuses_____
PRE/Body Sense_____
Notes_____

_____

Wednesday
Workout/Route_____
Mileage/Time/Pace_____
Focuses_____
PRE/Body Sense_____
Notes_____

_____

Thursday
Workout/Route_____
Mileage/Time/Pace_____
Focuses_____
PRE/Body Sense_____
Notes_____

_____

Friday
Workout/Route_____
Mileage/Time/Pace_____
Focuses_____
PRE/Body Sense_____
Notes_____

_____

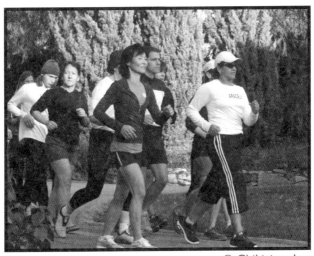

© ChiLiving,, Inc.

Saturday

Workout/Route _____

Mileage/Time/Pace _____

Focuses _____

PRE/Body Sense _____

Notes _____

_____

Sunday

Workout/Route _____

Mileage/Time/Pace _____

Focuses _____

PRE/Body Sense _____

Notes _____

_____

End-of-Week Review

Total Mileage/Time _____ Year-to-Date _____

Weight/BMI _____ Shoe A _____ Shoe B _____

Make a Choice and Move Forward _____

_____

_____

_____

Current Phase _____ Training Week # _____

Monday
Workout/Route _____
Mileage/Time/Pace _____
Focuses _____
PRE/Body Sense _____
Notes _____
_____

Tuesday
Workout/Route _____
Mileage/Time/Pace _____
Focuses _____
PRE/Body Sense _____
Notes _____
_____

Wednesday
Workout/Route _____
Mileage/Time/Pace _____
Focuses _____
PRE/Body Sense _____
Notes _____
_____

Thursday
Workout/Route _____
Mileage/Time/Pace _____
Focuses _____
PRE/Body Sense _____
Notes _____
_____

Friday
Workout/Route _____
Mileage/Time/Pace _____
Focuses _____
PRE/Body Sense _____
Notes _____
_____

Tip:
Imagine asphalt as a thin layer of ice and it will help you run with a very soft footstrike.

Saturday
Workout/Route _____
Mileage/Time/Pace _____
Focuses _____
PRE/Body Sense _____
Notes _____
_____

Sunday
Workout/Route _____
Mileage/Time/Pace _____
Focuses _____
PRE/Body Sense _____
Notes _____
_____

End-of-Week Review
Total Mileage/Time _____ Year-to-Date _____
Weight/BMI _____ Shoe A _____ Shoe B _____
Make a Choice and Move Forward _____
_____
_____
_____

Current Phase _____ Training Week # _____

Monday
Workout/Route _____
Mileage/Time/Pace _____
Focuses _____
PRE/Body Sense _____
Notes _____
_____

Tuesday
Workout/Route _____
Mileage/Time/Pace _____
Focuses _____
PRE/Body Sense _____
Notes _____
_____

Wednesday
Workout/Route _____
Mileage/Time/Pace _____
Focuses _____
PRE/Body Sense _____
Notes _____
_____

Thursday
Workout/Route _____
Mileage/Time/Pace _____
Focuses _____
PRE/Body Sense _____
Notes _____
_____

Friday
Workout/Route _____
Mileage/Time/Pace _____
Focuses _____
PRE/Body Sense _____
Notes _____
_____

> "Know your limits, but never stop trying to exceed them."
> – *Anonymous*

Saturday
Workout/Route _____
Mileage/Time/Pace _____
Focuses _____
PRE/Body Sense _____
Notes _____
_____

Sunday
Workout/Route _____
Mileage/Time/Pace _____
Focuses _____
PRE/Body Sense _____
Notes _____
_____

End-of-Week Review
Total Mileage/Time _____ Year-to-Date _____
Weight/BMI _____ Shoe A _____ Shoe B _____
Make a Choice and Move Forward _____
_____
_____
_____

Current Phase _____ Training Week # _____

Monday
Workout/Route _____

Mileage/Time/Pace _____

Focuses _____

PRE/Body Sense _____

Notes _____

_____

Tuesday
Workout/Route _____

Mileage/Time/Pace _____

Focuses _____

PRE/Body Sense _____

Notes _____

_____

Wednesday
Workout/Route _____

Mileage/Time/Pace _____

Focuses _____

PRE/Body Sense _____

Notes _____

_____

Thursday
Workout/Route _____

Mileage/Time/Pace _____

Focuses _____

PRE/Body Sense _____

Notes _____

_____

Friday
Workout/Route _____

Mileage/Time/Pace _____

Focuses _____

PRE/Body Sense _____

Notes _____

_____

Month _____ Week _____

> "There is more to life than increasing
> its speed."
> – Ghandi

Saturday
Workout/Route _____
Mileage/Time/Pace _____
Focuses _____
PRE/Body Sense _____
Notes _____
_____

Sunday
Workout/Route _____
Mileage/Time/Pace _____
Focuses _____
PRE/Body Sense _____
Notes _____
_____

End-of-Week Review
Total Mileage/Time _____ Year-to-Date _____
Weight/BMI _____ Shoe A _____ Shoe B _____
Make a Choice and Move Forward _____
_____
_____
_____

SUN	MON	TUE	WED	THU	FRI	SAT

"Learning is a treasure that will follow its owner everywhere. "

– Chinese Proverb

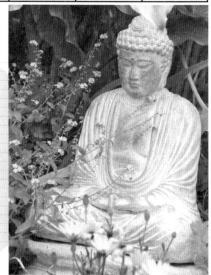

Dates:

Training Week #:

Weekly Goal:

Focus/Lesson:

Dates:

Training Week #:

Weekly Goal:

Focus/Lesson:

Dates:

Training Week #:

Weekly Goal:

Focus/Lesson:

Dates:

Training Week #:

Weekly Goal:

Focus/Lesson:

Dates:

Training Week #:

Weekly Goal:

Focus/Lesson:

Current Phase_____Training Week #_____

Monday
Workout/Route_____
Mileage/Time/Pace_____
Focuses_____
PRE/Body Sense_____
Notes_____
_____

Tuesday
Workout/Route_____
Mileage/Time/Pace_____
Focuses_____
PRE/Body Sense_____
Notes_____
_____

Wednesday
Workout/Route_____
Mileage/Time/Pace_____
Focuses_____
PRE/Body Sense_____
Notes_____
_____

Thursday
Workout/Route_____
Mileage/Time/Pace_____
Focuses_____
PRE/Body Sense_____
Notes_____
_____

Friday
Workout/Route_____
Mileage/Time/Pace_____
Focuses_____
PRE/Body Sense_____
Notes_____
_____

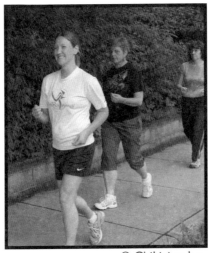

© ChiLiving, Inc.

Saturday
Workout/Route _____
Mileage/Time/Pace _____
Focuses _____
PRE/Body Sense _____
Notes _____

Sunday
Workout/Route _____
Mileage/Time/Pace _____
Focuses _____
PRE/Body Sense _____
Notes _____

End-of-Week Review
Total Mileage/Time _____ Year-to-Date _____
Weight/BMI _____ Shoe A _____ Shoe B _____
Make a Choice and Move Forward _____
_____
_____
_____

Current Phase_____ Training Week #_____

Monday
Workout/Route_____
Mileage/Time/Pace_____
Focuses_____
PRE/Body Sense_____
Notes_____
_____

Tuesday
Workout/Route_____
Mileage/Time/Pace_____
Focuses_____
PRE/Body Sense_____
Notes_____
_____

Wednesday
Workout/Route_____
Mileage/Time/Pace_____
Focuses_____
PRE/Body Sense_____
Notes_____
_____

Thursday
Workout/Route_____
Mileage/Time/Pace_____
Focuses_____
PRE/Body Sense_____
Notes_____
_____

Friday
Workout/Route_____
Mileage/Time/Pace_____
Focuses_____
PRE/Body Sense_____
Notes_____
_____

Month _____ Week _____

Tip:
Always eat a good protein meal
(meat, fish, poultry, tofu) after a
strenuous workout. It helps your
body to build and rebuild
muscle tissue.

Saturday
Workout/Route _____
Mileage/Time/Pace _____
Focuses _____
PRE/Body Sense _____
Notes _____
_____

Sunday
Workout/Route _____
Mileage/Time/Pace _____
Focuses _____
PRE/Body Sense _____
Notes _____
_____

End-of-Week Review
Total Mileage/Time _____ Year-to-Date _____
Weight/BMI _____ Shoe A _____ Shoe B _____
Make a Choice and Move Forward _____
_____
_____

Current Phase_____Training Week #_____

Monday
Workout/Route_____
Mileage/Time/Pace_____
Focuses_____
PRE/Body Sense_____
Notes_____

_____

Tuesday
Workout/Route_____
Mileage/Time/Pace_____
Focuses_____
PRE/Body Sense_____
Notes_____

_____

Wednesday
Workout/Route_____
Mileage/Time/Pace_____
Focuses_____
PRE/Body Sense_____
Notes_____

_____

Thursday
Workout/Route_____
Mileage/Time/Pace_____
Focuses_____
PRE/Body Sense_____
Notes_____

_____

Friday
Workout/Route_____
Mileage/Time/Pace_____
Focuses_____
PRE/Body Sense_____
Notes_____

_____

"Leap, and the net will appear."
– *Julie Cameron*

Saturday
Workout/Route _____
Mileage/Time/Pace _____
Focuses _____
PRE/Body Sense _____
Notes _____
_____

Sunday
Workout/Route _____
Mileage/Time/Pace _____
Focuses _____
PRE/Body Sense _____
Notes _____
_____

End-of-Week Review
Total Mileage/Time _____ Year-to-Date _____
Weight/BMI _____ Shoe A _____ Shoe B _____
Make a Choice and Move Forward _____
_____
_____
_____

Current Phase _____Training Week # _____

Monday
Workout/Route _____
Mileage/Time/Pace _____
Focuses _____
PRE/Body Sense _____
Notes _____

_____

Tuesday
Workout/Route _____
Mileage/Time/Pace _____
Focuses _____
PRE/Body Sense _____
Notes _____

_____

Wednesday
Workout/Route _____
Mileage/Time/Pace _____
Focuses _____
PRE/Body Sense _____
Notes _____

_____

Thursday
Workout/Route _____
Mileage/Time/Pace _____
Focuses _____
PRE/Body Sense _____
Notes _____

_____

Friday
Workout/Route _____
Mileage/Time/Pace _____
Focuses _____
PRE/Body Sense _____
Notes _____

_____

Tip:
You can check your lean when you run past a large glass storefront. Just don't get caught fixing your hair.

Saturday
Workout/Route _____
Mileage/Time/Pace _____
Focuses _____
PRE/Body Sense _____
Notes _____
_____

Sunday
Workout/Route _____
Mileage/Time/Pace _____
Focuses _____
PRE/Body Sense _____
Notes _____
_____

End-of-Week Review
Total Mileage/Time _____ Year-to-Date _____
Weight/BMI _____ Shoe A _____ Shoe B _____
Make a Choice and Move Forward _____
_____
_____
_____

Current Phase_____Training Week #_____

Monday
Workout/Route_____
Mileage/Time/Pace_____
Focuses_____
PRE/Body Sense_____
Notes_____
_____
_____

Tuesday
Workout/Route_____
Mileage/Time/Pace_____
Focuses_____
PRE/Body Sense_____
Notes_____
_____
_____

Wednesday
Workout/Route_____
Mileage/Time/Pace_____
Focuses_____
PRE/Body Sense_____
Notes_____
_____
_____

Thursday
Workout/Route_____
Mileage/Time/Pace_____
Focuses_____
PRE/Body Sense_____
Notes_____
_____
_____

Friday
Workout/Route_____
Mileage/Time/Pace_____
Focuses_____
PRE/Body Sense_____
Notes_____
_____
_____

Month _____ Week _____

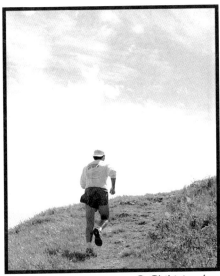

© ChiLiving, Inc.

Saturday
Workout/Route _____
Mileage/Time/Pace _____
Focuses _____
PRE/Body Sense _____
Notes _____
_____

Sunday
Workout/Route _____
Mileage/Time/Pace _____
Focuses _____
PRE/Body Sense _____
Notes _____
_____

End-of-Week Review
Total Mileage/Time _____ Year-to-Date _____
Weight/BMI _____ Shoe A _____ Shoe B _____
Make a Choice and Move Forward _____
_____
_____
_____

SUN	MON	TUE	WED	THU	FRI	SAT

"Success is getting what you want. Happiness is wanting what you get."

– Dale Carnagie

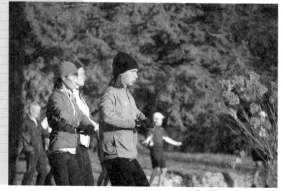

Dates:

Training Week #:

Weekly Goal:

Focus/Lesson:

Dates:

Training Week #:

Weekly Goal:

Focus/Lesson:

Dates:

Training Week #:

Weekly Goal:

Focus/Lesson:

Dates:

Training Week #:

Weekly Goal:

Focus/Lesson:

Dates:

Training Week #:

Weekly Goal:

Focus/Lesson:

Current Phase _____ Training Week # _____

Monday
Workout/Route _____

Mileage/Time/Pace _____

Focuses _____

PRE/Body Sense _____

Notes _____

_____

_____

Tuesday
Workout/Route _____

Mileage/Time/Pace _____

Focuses _____

PRE/Body Sense _____

Notes _____

_____

_____

Wednesday
Workout/Route _____

Mileage/Time/Pace _____

Focuses _____

PRE/Body Sense _____

Notes _____

_____

_____

Thursday
Workout/Route _____

Mileage/Time/Pace _____

Focuses _____

PRE/Body Sense _____

Notes _____

_____

_____

Friday
Workout/Route _____

Mileage/Time/Pace _____

Focuses _____

PRE/Body Sense _____

Notes _____

_____

_____

Tip:
You'll have a much better race if you're not standing around with your legs getting stale: Time your warm up to end at the start line right when the gun goes off, or do the knee-bending exercise in place to keep your legs warm.

Saturday
Workout/Route _____
Mileage/Time/Pace _____
Focuses _____
PRE/Body Sense _____
Notes _____
_____

Sunday
Workout/Route _____
Mileage/Time/Pace _____
Focuses _____
PRE/Body Sense _____
Notes _____
_____

End-of-Week Review
Total Mileage/Time _____Year-to-Date _____
Weight/BMI _____ Shoe A _____ Shoe B _____
Make a Choice and Move Forward _____
_____
_____

Current Phase _____ Training Week # _____

Monday
Workout/Route _____

Mileage/Time/Pace _____

Focuses _____

PRE/Body Sense _____

Notes _____

_____

Tuesday
Workout/Route _____

Mileage/Time/Pace _____

Focuses _____

PRE/Body Sense _____

Notes _____

_____

Wednesday
Workout/Route _____

Mileage/Time/Pace _____

Focuses _____

PRE/Body Sense _____

Notes _____

_____

Thursday
Workout/Route _____

Mileage/Time/Pace _____

Focuses _____

PRE/Body Sense _____

Notes _____

_____

Friday
Workout/Route _____

Mileage/Time/Pace _____

Focuses _____

PRE/Body Sense _____

Notes _____

_____

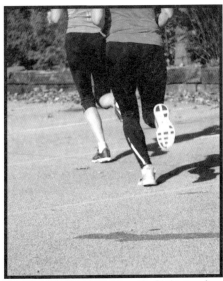

© ChiLiving, Inc.

Saturday
Workout/Route _____
Mileage/Time/Pace _____
Focuses _____
PRE/Body Sense _____
Notes _____
_____

Sunday
Workout/Route _____
Mileage/Time/Pace _____
Focuses _____
PRE/Body Sense _____
Notes _____
_____

End-of-Week Review
Total Mileage/Time _____ Year-to-Date _____
Weight/BMI _____ Shoe A _____ Shoe B _____
Make a Choice and Move Forward _____
_____
_____

Current Phase_____Training Week #_____

Monday
Workout/Route_____
Mileage/Time/Pace_____
Focuses_____
PRE/Body Sense_____
Notes_____
_____

Tuesday
Workout/Route_____
Mileage/Time/Pace_____
Focuses_____
PRE/Body Sense_____
Notes_____
_____

Wednesday
Workout/Route_____
Mileage/Time/Pace_____
Focuses_____
PRE/Body Sense_____
Notes_____
_____

Thursday
Workout/Route_____
Mileage/Time/Pace_____
Focuses_____
PRE/Body Sense_____
Notes_____
_____

Friday
Workout/Route_____
Mileage/Time/Pace_____
Focuses_____
PRE/Body Sense_____
Notes_____
_____

Tip:
When you're training for a race, practice your starting pace so that you know what to do on race day.

Saturday
Workout/Route _____

Mileage/Time/Pace _____

Focuses _____

PRE/Body Sense _____

Notes _____

_____

Sunday
Workout/Route _____

Mileage/Time/Pace _____

Focuses _____

PRE/Body Sense _____

Notes _____

_____

End-of-Week Review
Total Mileage/Time _____ Year-to-Date _____

Weight/BMI _____ Shoe A _____ Shoe B _____

Make a Choice and Move Forward _____

_____

_____

_____

Current Phase _____Training Week # _____

Monday
Workout/Route _____
Mileage/Time/Pace _____
Focuses _____
PRE/Body Sense _____
Notes _____
_____

Tuesday
Workout/Route _____
Mileage/Time/Pace _____
Focuses _____
PRE/Body Sense _____
Notes _____
_____

Wednesday
Workout/Route _____
Mileage/Time/Pace _____
Focuses _____
PRE/Body Sense _____
Notes _____
_____

Thursday
Workout/Route _____
Mileage/Time/Pace _____
Focuses _____
PRE/Body Sense _____
Notes _____
_____

Friday
Workout/Route _____
Mileage/Time/Pace _____
Focuses _____
PRE/Body Sense _____
Notes _____
_____

> "To have striven, to have made the effort, to have been true to certain ideals – this alone is worth the struggle."
> – *William Renn*

Saturday
Workout/Route ————————————————————
Mileage/Time/Pace ————————————————
Focuses ———————————————————————
PRE/Body Sense ————————————————————
Notes ————————————————————————

Sunday
Workout/Route ————————————————————
Mileage/Time/Pace ————————————————
Focuses ———————————————————————
PRE/Body Sense ————————————————————
Notes ————————————————————————

End-of-Week Review
Total Mileage/Time ————————————— Year-to-Date ————————
Weight/BMI ————————————— Shoe A ————— Shoe B —————
Make a Choice and Move Forward ——————————————————

Current Phase_____Training Week #_____

Monday
Workout/Route_____
Mileage/Time/Pace_____
Focuses_____
PRE/Body Sense_____
Notes_____
_____

Tuesday
Workout/Route_____
Mileage/Time/Pace_____
Focuses_____
PRE/Body Sense_____
Notes_____
_____

Wednesday
Workout/Route_____
Mileage/Time/Pace_____
Focuses_____
PRE/Body Sense_____
Notes_____
_____

Thursday
Workout/Route_____
Mileage/Time/Pace_____
Focuses_____
PRE/Body Sense_____
Notes_____
_____

Friday
Workout/Route_____
Mileage/Time/Pace_____
Focuses_____
PRE/Body Sense_____
Notes_____
_____

Month _____ Week _____

> "I have done my best: that is about all the philosophy of living one needs."
> – Lin-yutang

Saturday
Workout/Route _____
Mileage/Time/Pace _____
Focuses _____
PRE/Body Sense _____
Notes _____
_____

Sunday
Workout/Route _____
Mileage/Time/Pace _____
Focuses _____
PRE/Body Sense _____
Notes _____
_____

End-of-Week Review
Total Mileage/Time _____ Year-to-Date _____
Weight/BMI _____ Shoe A _____ Shoe B _____
Make a Choice and Move Forward _____
_____
_____
_____

SUN	MON	TUE	WED	THU	FRI	SAT

"The thing that is really hard, and really amazing, is giving up on being perfect and beginning the work of becoming yourself."

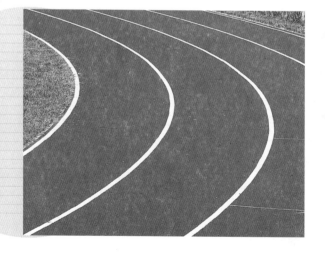

– Anna Quindlen

Dates:

Training Week #:

Weekly Goal:

Focus/Lesson:

Dates:

Training Week #:

Weekly Goal:

Focus/Lesson:

Dates:

Training Week #:

Weekly Goal:

Focus/Lesson:

Dates:

Training Week #:

Weekly Goal:

Focus/Lesson:

Dates:

Training Week #:

Weekly Goal:

Focus/Lesson:

Current Phase _____ Training Week # _____

Monday
Workout/Route _____

Mileage/Time/Pace _____

Focuses _____

PRE/Body Sense _____

Notes _____

_____

_____

Tuesday
Workout/Route _____

Mileage/Time/Pace _____

Focuses _____

PRE/Body Sense _____

Notes _____

_____

_____

Wednesday
Workout/Route _____

Mileage/Time/Pace _____

Focuses _____

PRE/Body Sense _____

Notes _____

_____

_____

Thursday
Workout/Route _____

Mileage/Time/Pace _____

Focuses _____

PRE/Body Sense _____

Notes _____

_____

_____

Friday
Workout/Route _____

Mileage/Time/Pace _____

Focuses _____

PRE/Body Sense _____

Notes _____

_____

_____

Tip:
Your body is just like a car that needs to downshift for the uphills. Do this by shortening your stride and using more arm swing.

Saturday
Workout/Route _____
Mileage/Time/Pace _____
Focuses _____
PRE/Body Sense _____
Notes _____
_____

Sunday
Workout/Route _____
Mileage/Time/Pace _____
Focuses _____
PRE/Body Sense _____
Notes _____
_____

End-of-Week Review
Total Mileage/Time _____ Year-to-Date _____
Weight/BMI _____ Shoe A _____ Shoe B _____
Make a Choice and Move Forward _____
_____
_____
_____

Monday
Workout/Route————————————————————————————
Mileage/Time/Pace—————————————————————————
Focuses——————————————————————————————
PRE/Body Sense————————————————————————————
Notes—————————————————————————————————

Tuesday
Workout/Route————————————————————————————
Mileage/Time/Pace—————————————————————————
Focuses——————————————————————————————
PRE/Body Sense————————————————————————————
Notes—————————————————————————————————

Wednesday
Workout/Route————————————————————————————
Mileage/Time/Pace—————————————————————————
Focuses——————————————————————————————
PRE/Body Sense————————————————————————————
Notes—————————————————————————————————

Thursday
Workout/Route————————————————————————————
Mileage/Time/Pace—————————————————————————
Focuses——————————————————————————————
PRE/Body Sense————————————————————————————
Notes—————————————————————————————————

Friday
Workout/Route————————————————————————————
Mileage/Time/Pace—————————————————————————
Focuses——————————————————————————————
PRE/Body Sense————————————————————————————
Notes—————————————————————————————————

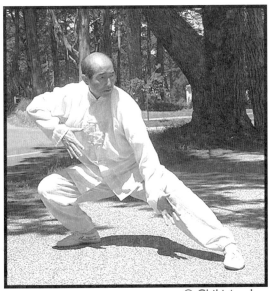

© ChiLiving, Inc.

Saturday
Workout/Route _____
Mileage/Time/Pace _____
Focuses _____
PRE/Body Sense _____
Notes _____
_____

Sunday
Workout/Route _____
Mileage/Time/Pace _____
Focuses _____
PRE/Body Sense _____
Notes _____
_____

End-of-Week Review
Total Mileage/Time _____ Year-to-Date _____
Weight/BMI _____ Shoe A _____ Shoe B _____
Make a Choice and Move Forward _____
_____
_____
_____

Current Phase _____ Training Week # _____

Monday
Workout/Route _____
Mileage/Time/Pace _____
Focuses _____
PRE/Body Sense _____
Notes _____
_____
_____

Tuesday
Workout/Route _____
Mileage/Time/Pace _____
Focuses _____
PRE/Body Sense _____
Notes _____
_____
_____

Wednesday
Workout/Route _____
Mileage/Time/Pace _____
Focuses _____
PRE/Body Sense _____
Notes _____
_____
_____

Thursday
Workout/Route _____
Mileage/Time/Pace _____
Focuses _____
PRE/Body Sense _____
Notes _____
_____
_____

Friday
Workout/Route _____
Mileage/Time/Pace _____
Focuses _____
PRE/Body Sense _____
Notes _____
_____

Month _____ Week _____

Tip:
Diet and nutrition are very important.
Make sure you're getting all of the vitamins
and minerals that you need through your diet
or from a good multi-vitamin
and mineral supplement.

Saturday
Workout/Route _____
Mileage/Time/Pace _____
Focuses _____
PRE/Body Sense _____
Notes _____
_____

Sunday
Workout/Route _____
Mileage/Time/Pace _____
Focuses _____
PRE/Body Sense _____
Notes _____
_____

End-of-Week Review
Total Mileage/Time _____ Year-to-Date _____
Weight/BMI _____ Shoe A _____ Shoe B _____
Make a Choice and Move Forward _____
_____
_____
_____

Monday
Workout/Route_____
Mileage/Time/Pace_____
Focuses_____
PRE/Body Sense_____
Notes_____

_____

Tuesday
Workout/Route_____
Mileage/Time/Pace_____
Focuses_____
PRE/Body Sense_____
Notes_____

_____

Wednesday
Workout/Route_____
Mileage/Time/Pace_____
Focuses_____
PRE/Body Sense_____
Notes_____

_____

Thursday
Workout/Route_____
Mileage/Time/Pace_____
Focuses_____
PRE/Body Sense_____
Notes_____

_____

Friday
Workout/Route_____
Mileage/Time/Pace_____
Focuses_____
PRE/Body Sense_____
Notes_____

_____

> "Nothing in life is to be feared. It is only to be understood."
> – *Marie Curie*

Saturday
Workout/Route _____

Mileage/Time/Pace _____

Focuses _____

PRE/Body Sense _____

Notes _____

_____

Sunday
Workout/Route _____

Mileage/Time/Pace _____

Focuses _____

PRE/Body Sense _____

Notes _____

_____

End-of-Week Review
Total Mileage/Time _____ Year-to-Date _____

Weight/BMI _____ Shoe A _____ Shoe B _____

Make a Choice and Move Forward _____

_____

_____

_____

Current Phase_____Training Week #_____

Monday
Workout/Route_____
Mileage/Time/Pace_____
Focuses_____
PRE/Body Sense_____
Notes_____
_____

Tuesday
Workout/Route_____
Mileage/Time/Pace_____
Focuses_____
PRE/Body Sense_____
Notes_____
_____

Wednesday
Workout/Route_____
Mileage/Time/Pace_____
Focuses_____
PRE/Body Sense_____
Notes_____
_____

Thursday
Workout/Route_____
Mileage/Time/Pace_____
Focuses_____
PRE/Body Sense_____
Notes_____
_____

Friday
Workout/Route_____
Mileage/Time/Pace_____
Focuses_____
PRE/Body Sense_____
Notes_____
_____

> "Joy comes from using your potential."
> – *Will Schultz*

Saturday
Workout/Route _____
Mileage/Time/Pace _____
Focuses _____
PRE/Body Sense _____
Notes _____
_____

Sunday
Workout/Route _____
Mileage/Time/Pace _____
Focuses _____
PRE/Body Sense _____
Notes _____
_____

End-of-Week Review
Total Mileage/Time _____ Year-to-Date _____
Weight/BMI _____ Shoe A _____ Shoe B _____
Make a Choice and Move Forward _____
_____
_____
_____

SUN	MON	TUE	WED	THU	FRI	SAT

"How wonderful
it is that nobody
need wait a
single moment
before starting
to improve the
world."

– Anne Frank

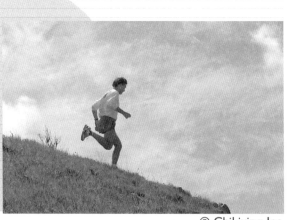

Dates:

Training Week #:

Weekly Goal:

Focus/Lesson:

Dates:

Training Week #:

Weekly Goal:

Focus/Lesson:

Dates:

Training Week #:

Weekly Goal:

Focus/Lesson:

Dates:

Training Week #:

Weekly Goal:

Focus/Lesson:

Dates:

Training Week #:

Weekly Goal:

Focus/Lesson:

Current Phase _____ Training Week # _____

Monday
Workout/Route _____
Mileage/Time/Pace _____
Focuses _____
PRE/Body Sense _____
Notes _____
_____

Tuesday
Workout/Route _____
Mileage/Time/Pace _____
Focuses _____
PRE/Body Sense _____
Notes _____
_____

Wednesday
Workout/Route _____
Mileage/Time/Pace _____
Focuses _____
PRE/Body Sense _____
Notes _____
_____

Thursday
Workout/Route _____
Mileage/Time/Pace _____
Focuses _____
PRE/Body Sense _____
Notes _____
_____

Friday
Workout/Route _____
Mileage/Time/Pace _____
Focuses _____
PRE/Body Sense _____
Notes _____
_____

Tip:
Stay tall by pushing up the sky.
Imagine that the crown of your head
is supporting the clouds.

Saturday
Workout/Route _____
Mileage/Time/Pace _____
Focuses _____
PRE/Body Sense _____
Notes _____

Sunday
Workout/Route _____
Mileage/Time/Pace _____
Focuses _____
PRE/Body Sense _____
Notes _____

End-of-Week Review
Total Mileage/Time _____ Year-to-Date _____
Weight/BMI _____ Shoe A _____ Shoe B _____
Make a Choice and Move Forward _____

Current Phase _____ Training Week # _____

Monday
Workout/Route _____

Mileage/Time/Pace _____

Focuses _____

PRE/Body Sense _____

Notes _____

_____

Tuesday
Workout/Route _____

Mileage/Time/Pace _____

Focuses _____

PRE/Body Sense _____

Notes _____

_____

Wednesday
Workout/Route _____

Mileage/Time/Pace _____

Focuses _____

PRE/Body Sense _____

Notes _____

_____

Thursday
Workout/Route _____

Mileage/Time/Pace _____

Focuses _____

PRE/Body Sense _____

Notes _____

_____

Friday
Workout/Route _____

Mileage/Time/Pace _____

Focuses _____

PRE/Body Sense _____

Notes _____

_____

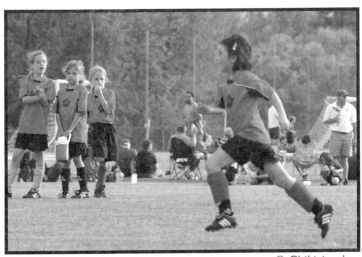

© ChiLiving, Inc.

Saturday
Workout/Route _____
Mileage/Time/Pace _____
Focuses _____
PRE/Body Sense _____
Notes _____
_____

Sunday
Workout/Route _____
Mileage/Time/Pace _____
Focuses _____
PRE/Body Sense _____
Notes _____
_____

End-of-Week Review
Total Mileage/Time _____ Year-to-Date _____
Weight/BMI _____ Shoe A _____ Shoe B _____
Make a Choice and Move Forward _____
_____
_____
_____

Current Phase——————————————Training Week #——————

Monday
Workout/Route————————————————————
Mileage/Time/Pace————————————————
Focuses————————————————————————
PRE/Body Sense—————————————————
Notes—————————————————————————

_____

Tuesday
Workout/Route————————————————————
Mileage/Time/Pace————————————————
Focuses————————————————————————
PRE/Body Sense—————————————————
Notes—————————————————————————

_____

Wednesday
Workout/Route————————————————————
Mileage/Time/Pace————————————————
Focuses————————————————————————
PRE/Body Sense—————————————————
Notes—————————————————————————

_____

Thursday
Workout/Route————————————————————
Mileage/Time/Pace————————————————
Focuses————————————————————————
PRE/Body Sense—————————————————
Notes—————————————————————————

_____

Friday
Workout/Route————————————————————
Mileage/Time/Pace————————————————
Focuses————————————————————————
PRE/Body Sense—————————————————
Notes—————————————————————————

_____

Month _____ Week _____

Tip:
Remember the purpose of
Long Slow Distance runs: Done
correctly, they build aerobic
capacity, increasing capillary
beds in your lungs.

Saturday
Workout/Route _____
Mileage/Time/Pace _____
Focuses _____
PRE/Body Sense _____
Notes _____
_____

Sunday
Workout/Route _____
Mileage/Time/Pace _____
Focuses _____
PRE/Body Sense _____
Notes _____
_____

End-of-Week Review
Total Mileage/Time _____ Year-to-Date _____
Weight/BMI _____ Shoe A _____ Shoe B _____
Make a Choice and Move Forward _____
_____
_____
_____

Current Phase _____ Training Week # _____

Monday
Workout/Route _____
Mileage/Time/Pace _____
Focuses _____
PRE/Body Sense _____
Notes _____
_____

Tuesday
Workout/Route _____
Mileage/Time/Pace _____
Focuses _____
PRE/Body Sense _____
Notes _____
_____

Wednesday
Workout/Route _____
Mileage/Time/Pace _____
Focuses _____
PRE/Body Sense _____
Notes _____
_____

Thursday
Workout/Route _____
Mileage/Time/Pace _____
Focuses _____
PRE/Body Sense _____
Notes _____
_____

Friday
Workout/Route _____
Mileage/Time/Pace _____
Focuses _____
PRE/Body Sense _____
Notes _____
_____

> "Most of the shadows of this life
> are caused by our standing
> in our own sunshine."
> – *Ralph Waldo Emerson*

Saturday
Workout/Route _____
Mileage/Time/Pace _____
Focuses _____
PRE/Body Sense _____
Notes _____
_____

Sunday
Workout/Route _____
Mileage/Time/Pace _____
Focuses _____
PRE/Body Sense _____
Notes _____
_____

End-of-Week Review
Total Mileage/Time _____ Year-to-Date _____
Weight/BMI _____ Shoe A _____ Shoe B _____
Make a Choice and Move Forward _____
_____
_____
_____

Current Phase _____ Training Week # _____

Monday
Workout/Route _____
Mileage/Time/Pace _____
Focuses _____
PRE/Body Sense _____
Notes _____
_____

Tuesday
Workout/Route _____
Mileage/Time/Pace _____
Focuses _____
PRE/Body Sense _____
Notes _____
_____

Wednesday
Workout/Route _____
Mileage/Time/Pace _____
Focuses _____
PRE/Body Sense _____
Notes _____
_____

Thursday
Workout/Route _____
Mileage/Time/Pace _____
Focuses _____
PRE/Body Sense _____
Notes _____
_____

Friday
Workout/Route _____
Mileage/Time/Pace _____
Focuses _____
PRE/Body Sense _____
Notes _____
_____

Tip:
Get a training partner and use each other as inspiration for staying with your own individual programs.

Saturday
Workout/Route _____
Mileage/Time/Pace _____
Focuses _____
PRE/Body Sense _____
Notes _____
_____

Sunday
Workout/Route _____
Mileage/Time/Pace _____
Focuses _____
PRE/Body Sense _____
Notes _____
_____

End-of-Week Review
Total Mileage/Time _____ Year-to-Date _____
Weight/BMI _____ Shoe A _____ Shoe B _____
Make a Choice and Move Forward _____
_____
_____

APPENDIX A:
Vision, Goals and Assessments

Vision and Goals

Create a vision for yourself. This vision can be health related, fitness related, or even all-encompassing of your life, your health *and* your fitness. Whatever your vision is, take the time to think about it and write it down in the space below.

Write down specific goals that will help you accomplish your vision. Whatever your goals may be, please remember to make them realistic, manageable and challenging in a healthy way. They can be as specific as "Run a marathon" or as general as "Feel fit and lose weight."

_____

_____

_____

_____

_____

_____

_____

_____

_____

_____

_____

_____

_____

_____

_____

_____

Personal Assessments

Chi Running and Chi Walking help you learn to listen to your body and make adjustments to correct any source of discomfort or inefficient movement. Making regular assessments of your physical and psychological/emotional states gives you a better understanding of how your mind can direct your body and how your body will respond.

Physical Assessment – Are you happy with your overall weight and health? Do you have any health or physical concerns you need to take into consideration? Evaluate your overall health and energy level. Record your age, weight and blood pressure below.

Resting Heart Rate

It's helpful to know your Resting Heart Rate (RHR) and check it on a regular basis. To determine your RHR, check it before getting out of bed. Count the number of beats in 15 seconds by pressing your pointer and middle finger on your neck beneath your lower jaw, then multiply by four. As you get into better shape from your training, you may find your RHR gets lower, which is good news.

Maximum Aerobic Heart Rate

Another important statistic to be aware of is your maximum aerobic heart rate. To determine your maximum aerobic heart rate, subtract your age from 180 (180 – age). Your maximum aerobic heart rate should feel like a 7 on a scale of 1-10 (see the introduction for more on PRE [Perceived Rate of Exertion]). If you train and exercise within your aerobic heart rate (PRE 5-6), you'll eventually be able to move faster with less overall effort. You can use a heart rate monitor to keep track of your heart rate during workouts, or measure it using your pointer and middle fingers, as described above.

Psychological/Emotional Assessment – Any exercise routine is 10% physical and 90% power of the mind. Be aware of the thoughts that will enhance your exercising and training as well as the thoughts that might undermine your efforts. Put yourself on a "diet of the mind" and focus on the thoughts that are supportive of your vision and goals. Write down the qualities and characteristics you possess that will help you maintain healthy, lifelong habits. Have a plan to overcome the obstacles that your mind may create on your path to success.

_____

_____

_____

_____

_____

_____

_____

_____

_____

_____

_____

_____

_____

_____

_____

_____

_____

_____

_____

_____

_____

_____

_____

APPENDIX B:
Charting Your Progress

The following pages allow you to monitor and graph your weekly progress of several essential exercise components: distance, weight and Time Trial (time or average pace per mile).

Please see the next page for an example of how to use this chart. We have included a scale and units for each of the y-axes: distance (miles), weight (pounds) and Time Trial (minutes).

EXAMPLE

Mileage / Weight / Time Trial Chart

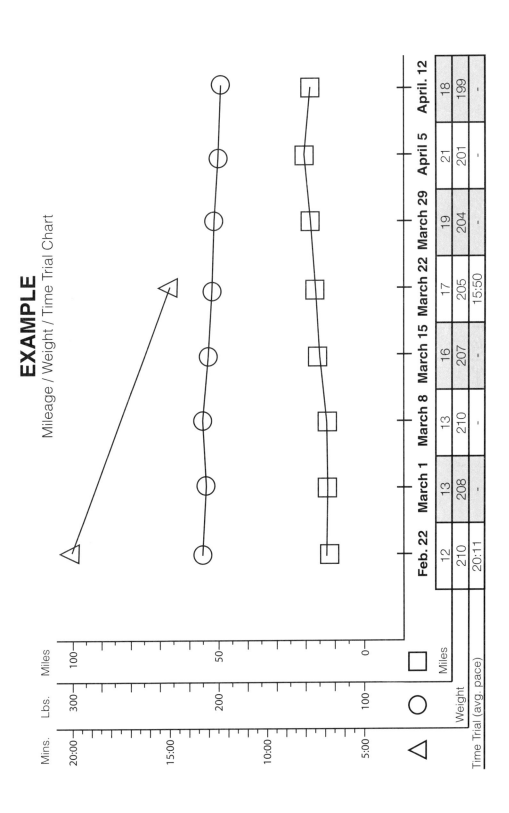

	Feb. 22	March 1	March 8	March 15	March 22	March 29	April 5	April. 12
Miles	12	13	13	16	17	19	21	18
Weight	210	208	210	207	205	204	201	199
Time Trial (avg. pace)	20:11	-	-	-	15:50	-	-	-

Weeks 1-8
Mileage / Weight / Time Trial Chart

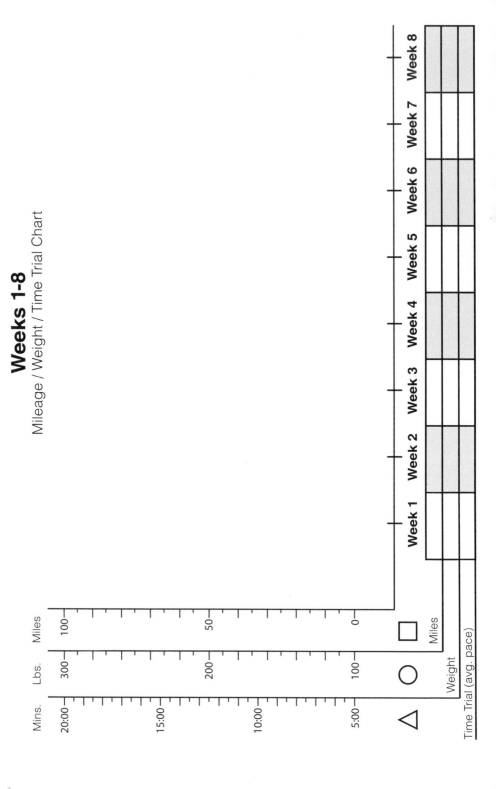

Weeks 9-16

Mileage / Weight / Time Trial Chart

	Week 9	Week 10	Week 11	Week 12	Week 13	Week 14	Week 15	Week 16
Miles □								
Weight ○								
Time Trial (avg. pace) △								

Miles (0–100)
Lbs. (100–300)
Mins. (5:00–20:00)

Weeks 17-24
Mileage / Weight / Time Trial Chart

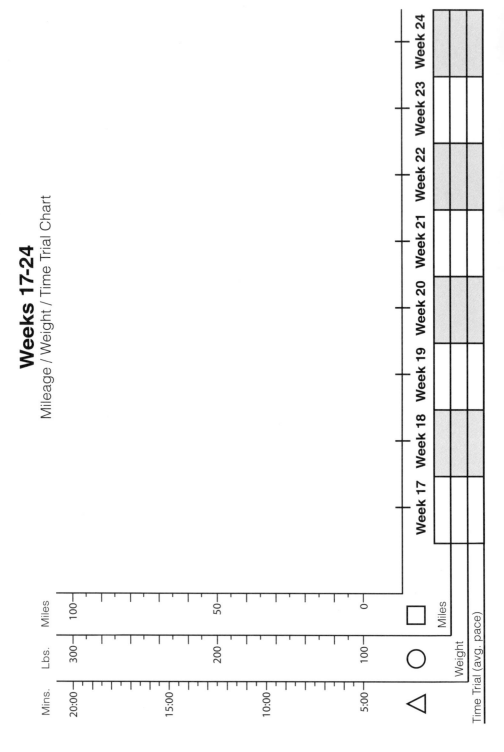

	Week 17	Week 18	Week 19	Week 20	Week 21	Week 22	Week 23	Week 24

□ Miles

○ Weight

△ Time Trial (avg. pace)

Miles — 100, 50, 0

Lbs. — 300, 200, 100

Mins. — 20:00, 15:00, 10:00, 5:00

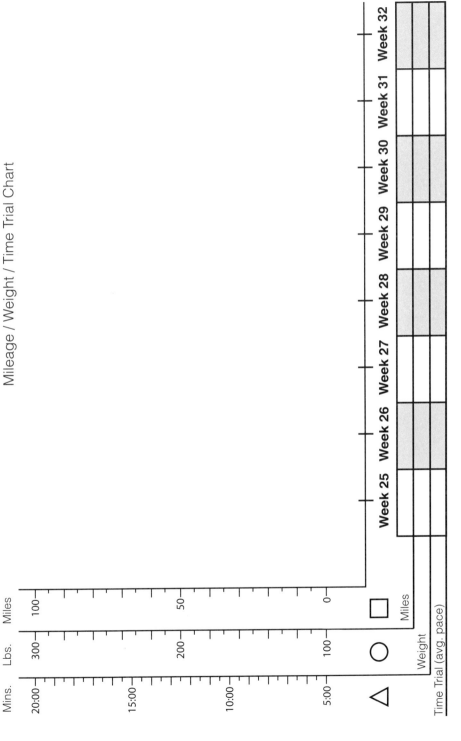

Weeks 25-32

Mileage / Weight / Time Trial Chart

Weeks 33-40

Mileage / Weight / Time Trial Chart

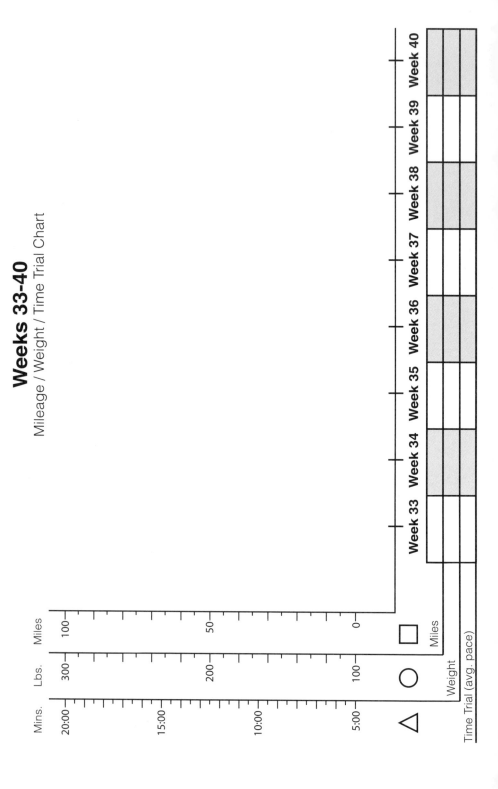

Weeks 41-48

Mileage / Weight / Time Trial Chart

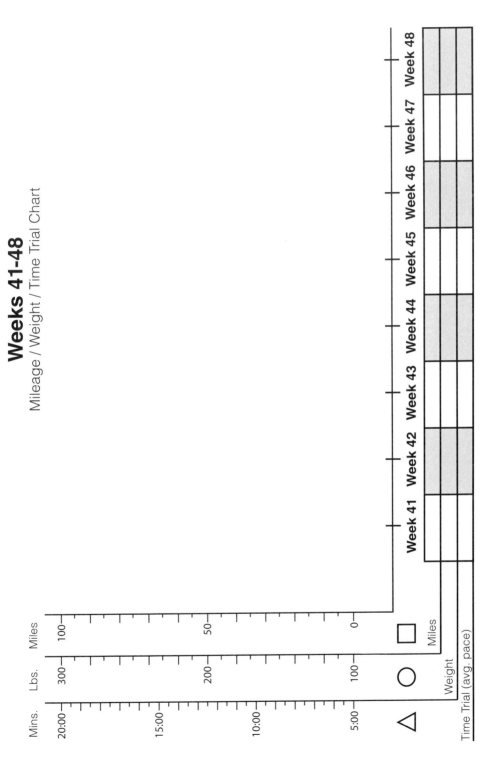

Weeks 49-52 / Next Year's Weeks 1-4
Mileage / Weight / Time Trial Chart

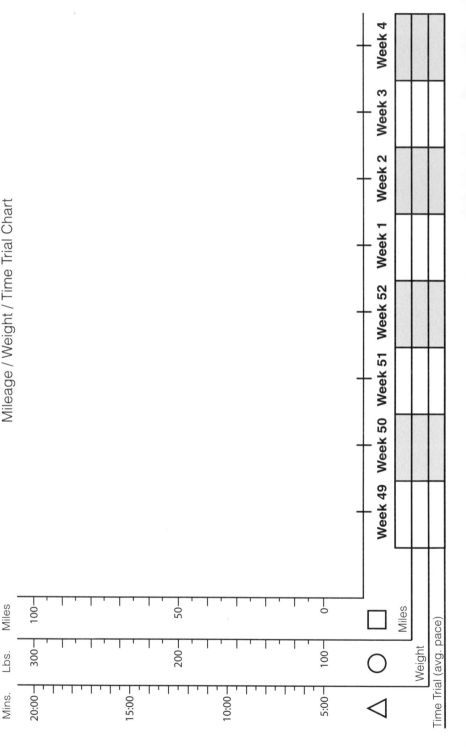

APPENDIX C:
ChiWalking Exercise Guide

The chart below helps walkers determine ideal cadence and PRE for particular types of workouts.

Each zone (type of walk) has its own ideal cadence (steps per minute) and Perceived Rate of Exertion (PRE). As with any kind of activity, be sure to consult your health practitioner before beginning any exercise program.

Zone	Cadence	PRE
Warm-up/Cool Down	55-65	2-3
Aerobic	60-70	4-5
Fitness/Weight Release	65-75	5-7
Cardio	70-80	8-9

Zones

Warm-up/Cool Down: At the beginning of each workout, you should transition gradually from a resting heart rate (RHR) into an elevated heart rate. The warm-up/cool down zone is designed to both "warm-up" and "cool down" your body before and after each workout. Ten minutes for both warm-up and cool down are ideal.

Aerobic: A great zone for building your aerobic capacity and for overall health and weight maintenance.

Fitness/Weight Release: If you're looking to lose weight, tone your muscles or increase your level of fitness, this is the best zone. Most effective when done for 30 plus minutes, especially for people on a weight-loss program. When you exercise for over 30 minutes, your body burns more body fat and less glycogen (sugar) and begins to rid the body of excess weight.

Cardio: This zone is best for people with a healthy weight. Cardio workouts really work your heart and lungs together, strengthening both. If you like to sweat, this zone is great! Remember that cardio workouts are generally shorter in length than aerobic or fitness walks. Warm-up and cool down are very important for cardio workouts.

Cadence/SPM

Cadence and SPM (Strides per Minute) are interchangeable terms that identify the number of steps taken by each foot during a 60-second period. For example, the Warm-Up/Cool Down zone suggests a cadence of 55-65. This means that over the course of 1 minute (60 seconds), each foot would take 55-65 steps.

We highly encourage walkers to use a metronome to help maintain correct cadence. Please see our website for more information or to order a metronome.

PRE

Perceived Rate of Exertion (PRE) is the amount of energy expenditure your body is making at any given moment. The numbers associated with PRE range from 1-10, 1 being no effort at all, 10 being the most effort possible. We encourage you to Body Sense your PRE and become familiar with how each level of exertion feels in your body.

You can also keep track of your PRE by measuring your heart rate. Please see Appendix A for more information about aerobic heart rate measurement and how it relates to PRE.

APPENDIX D:
ChiRunning and ChiWalking Focuses

	ChiRunning	ChiWalking
Posture		
Align your feet and legs	☑	☑
Soften your knees	☑	☑
Balance your feet (left/right, front/back, inside/outside)	☑	☑
Lengthen the back of your neck	☑	☑
Level your pelvis	☑	☑
Relax your glutes	☑	☑
Create your Column (shoulders, hips, ankles aligned)	☑	☑
Feel your feet at the bottom of your Column	☑	☑
One-legged posture stance	☑	☑
The "C" Shape	☑	☑
Feel your Column supporting each stride	☑	☐
Relax everything but your lower abs	☑	☑
Lean		
Three steps to engage lean	☑	☐
Lean from your hips	☐	☑
Relax lower legs and ankles	☑	☑
Lengthen the back of your neck and lead with your forehead	☑	☑
Lean from your ankles	☑	☐

Lean (continued)		
Shoulders ahead of your feet	☑	☑
Balance in the "window of lean"	☑	☐
Feel your lower abs and obliques engage more as you lean more	☑	☐
Lead with upper body, feet will follow	☑	☑
Your lean is your gas pedal	☑	☐
Lower Body: Legs		
Start off with short stride	☑	☑
Let your legs swing to the rear	☑	☑
Let your hip swing back with your leg	☑	☑
Rotate legs medially (toward your midline) to point feet forward	☑	☑
Knee straight at end of stride	☐	☑
Lower Body: Lower Legs		
Bend your knees	☑	☐
Limp lower legs: calves, shins, ankles, feet, toes	☑	☑
Heels up/knees down	☑	☐
Soften knees	☑	☑
Passive lower legs	☑	☑
Lift ankles	☑	☑
Feet point forward	☑	☑
Circular feet with wheels at the ends of your legs	☑	☐

Lower Body: Lower Legs (continued)		
Peel foot off the ground	☑	☑
Midfoot strike	☑	☐
Land on front of heel, roll forward	☐	☑
Lower Body: Pelvic Rotation		
Feel your Pivot Point at T12/L1	☑	☑
Level your pelvis	☑	☑
Allow pelvic rotation to happen	☑	☑
Rotate entire lower body below Pivot Point	☑	☑
Upper Body: Arm Swing		
Bend your elbows to 90° (don't pump)	☑	☐
Elbows 90° to 180°, depending on speed	☐	☑
Curl fingers, thumbs on top; relax hands	☑	☑
Hands always held above your waistline	☑	☐
Hands don't cross your center-line	☑	☑
Swing elbows to the rear	☑	☑
Shoulders fall forward	☑	☐
Upper Body: Head, Neck & Shoulders		
Keep shoulders low and relaxed	☑	☑
Shoulders always face forward	☑	☑
Lengthen back of neck; lengthen spine	☑	☑
Lead with your forehead, drop your chin	☑	☑
Y'chi directs energy forward through the eyes	☑	☑

Upper Body: Breathing

	🏃	🚶
Belly-breathe – Exhale through mouth by pulling your belly in, Inhale through nose, expanding your belly	☑	☑
Match breath rate to cadence: exhale for two steps, inhale for one	☑	☐
Nose-breathe if possible	☑	☑

Cadence

If your current cadence is below 85 spm, start there and increase cadence by one stride per minute each week until you reach 85	☑	☐
Cadence always stays the same	☑	☐
Cadence increases with speed	☐	☑

APPENDIX E: Race Log

Date	Event	Distance	Time	Pace	AG Place	Overall
Notes:						
Notes:						
Notes:						
Notes:						
Notes:						
Notes:						
Notes:						
Notes:						
Notes:						
Notes:						
Notes:						
Notes:						
Notes:						

Date	Event	Distance	Time	Pace	AG Place	Overall

Notes:

Notes:

Notes:

Notes:

Notes:

Notes:

Notes:

Notes:

Notes:

Notes:

Notes:

Notes:

Notes:

APPENDIX F:
Unit Conversions

Miles to Kilometers

Miles	Km	Miles	Km	Miles	Km
1	1.6	10	16.09	19	30.57
2	3.21	11	17.07	20	32.18
3	4.82	12	19.3	21	33.17
4	6.43	13	20.92	22	35.4
5	8.04	14	22.53	23	37.01
6	9.65	15	24.13	24	38.62
7	11.26	16	25.74	25	40.23
8	12.87	17	27.35	26	41.84
9	14.48	18	28.96	27	43.45

Kilometers to Miles

Km	Miles	Km	Miles
1	0.62	45	27.9
5	3.1	50	31
10	6.2	55	34.1
15	9.3	60	37.2
20	12.4	65	40.3
25	15.5	70	43.4
30	18.6	80	49.7
35	21.7	90	55.9
40	24.8	100	62.1

Additional training support and insights:

ChiRunning.com | *ChiWalking*.com

Visit us on the Web at ChiRunning.com or ChiWalking.com:

Chi Running and Chi Walking books and products, fitness watches, metronomes, apparel and more!

Free e-Newsletter • Ask the Expert Bulletin Board
A vast library of free, informative articles

Call Toll-Free: 1-866-327-7867